A History of Medicine in South West Durham

A.J.A. Ferguson, D.T. Prescott, F. Robertson

ISBN 0-9515068-0-3

Published by The South West Durham Health Authority, 1989
Printed by: Blamire Printers Ltd., Ferryhill, Co. Durham.

CONTENTS

ILLUSTRATIONS

Foreword

by

Mrs. Erika R. Wallis, B.Sc.

Chairman, South West Durham Health Authority

It gives me great pleasure to write the foreword for a book that I have watched grow from the germ of an idea into a fascinating account which I found difficult to put down.

The idea was first given to me by Dr. Bernard Walsh, Dr. Frank Robertson's successor and the first Physican with Special Responsibility for the Elderly at Bishop Auckland General Hospital.

We had hoped to publish the book to mark the 40th Anniversary of the National Health Service but the enormous amount of material generously supplied by so many people made the task greater than anticipated.

I should like to express, on behalf of South West Durham Health Authority, my thanks to the authors for the amount of time and effort they have given to the research and writing and above all for their generosity in allowing the profits to be used for patient care, also to all who have made this work such a wonderful collaborative effort.

The authors, through their long experience of caring for the sick in South West Durham, were able to highlight the great improvement in the care of the patients and in the social conditions. These improvements — not achieved without some struggle and strife — were brought about partly by legislation, partly by scientific progress, but would not have been possible without the dedication of the people who worked and still work in the service at all levels.

The book will be of interest not only to the people who regard the National Health Service in South West Durham as their service, but also to researchers into local history and the history of medicine.

I hope many people will show their appreciation by buying this book.

Erika Wallis

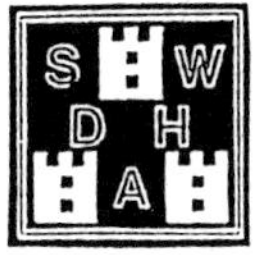

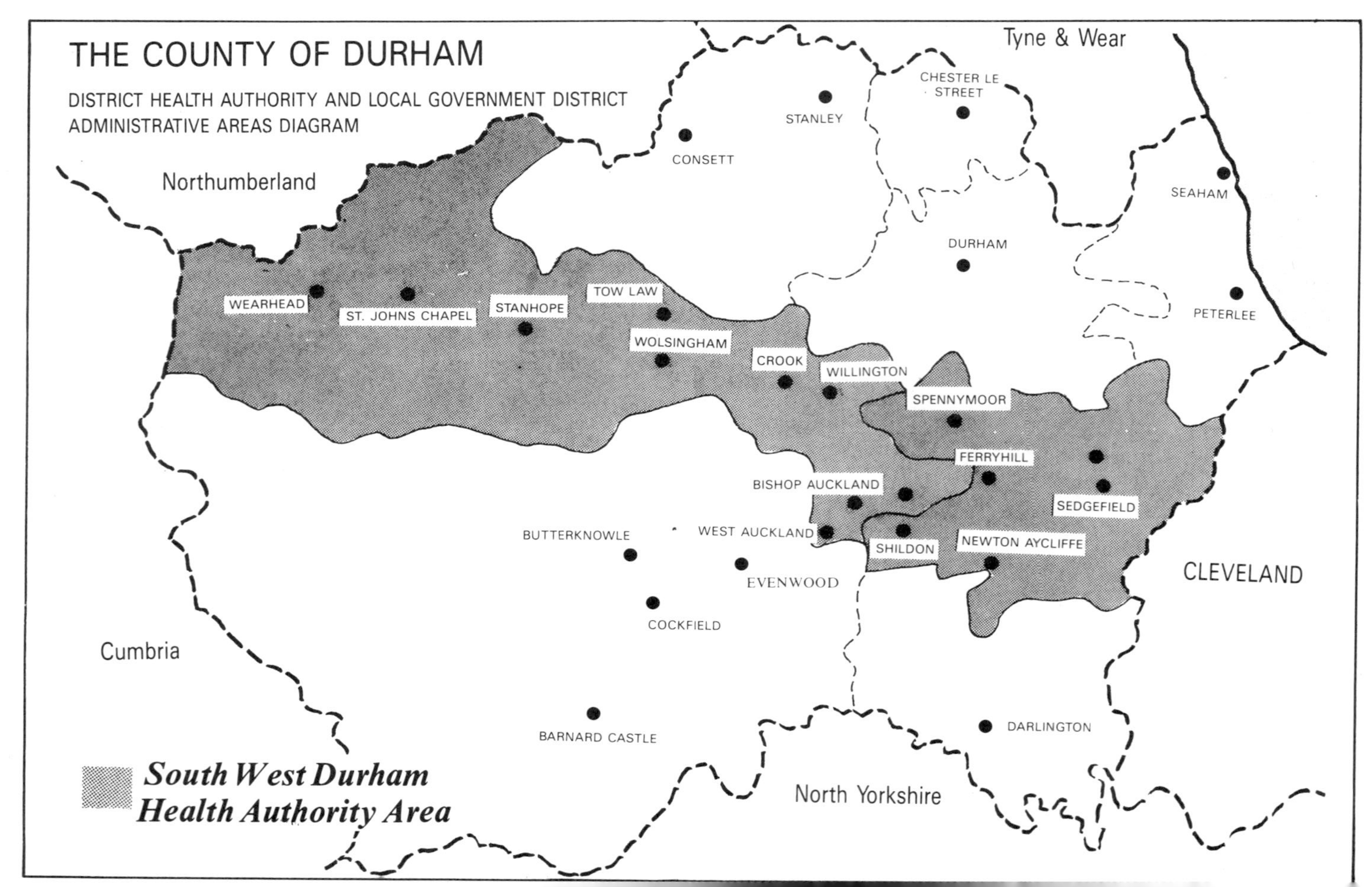
THE COUNTY OF DURHAM
DISTRICT HEALTH AUTHORITY AND LOCAL GOVERNMENT DISTRICT
ADMINISTRATIVE AREAS DIAGRAM
Northumberland
Tyne & Wear
CONSETT
STANLEY
CHESTER LE STREET
SEAHAM
DURHAM
PETERLEE
WEARHEAD
ST. JOHNS CHAPEL
STANHOPE
TOW LAW
WOLSINGHAM
CROOK
WILLINGTON
SPENNYMOOR
FERRYHILL
BISHOP AUCKLAND
SEDGEFIELD
WEST AUCKLAND
SHILDON
NEWTON AYCLIFFE
BUTTERKNOWLE
EVENWOOD
COCKFIELD
CLEVELAND
Cumbria
BARNARD CASTLE
DARLINGTON
North Yorkshire
South West Durham
Health Authority Area

ACKNOWLEDGEMENTS

Many of the contributors to this book have taken a great deal of time and trouble researching their practice and family histories, whilst others have drawn on their recollections as partners, assistants, receptionists, nurses, and patients. In addition we have had the good fortune to have access to family photographs, to photographs of Bishop Auckland General Hospital, and to the records of the old N.H.I. Committee of County Durham. Our thanks go to everyone who has helped us in one way or another, namely: Dr G. Adams, Dr G. Adan, Mrs Janet Alsted (Dr Janet Pope). Dr J.A. Anderson, Prof J.R. Anderson, Mr Anido K. Banerjee, Dr H. Bannerman, Dr K. Beveridge, Mrs Edith Botcherby, Dr E. Brauer, Dr B. Chamberlain, Dr A.I.A. Charlton, Dr J. Clark, Dr M. Clay, Mrs Norma Clennell, Dr J. Corrigan, Dr A.H. Dawes, Dr N. Deytrikh, Dr Patricia Downes, Mr G. Espiner (Administrator, Durham F.P.C.) Dr G.L. Ferguson, Dr. E.A. Fox, Mr Derek Foster M.P., Dr I. Fuller, Mrs Nancy Goldsbrough S.R.N., N.D.N. Cert., Dr R.P. Graham, Dr R.H. Grainger. Mrs Dorothy Halford, Mr H.S. Hamilton, Dr M.J. Harbinson, Mrs. Edith Hogarth S.R.N.S.C.M., Mr B. Hunt, Dr Maryan Huntridge, Dr W.D. Kerr, Mrs Jean Jamieson, Mr J. Land, Mrs Margaret Lodge, Mr R. Lewis, Dr I.G. Lloyd, Mrs. Margaret Markham S.R.N. H.V. Cert. Mr A.B.K. McCullagh, Mr S. McGreevy, Mrs Kathleen MacMillan, Dr A. McQueen, Mrs Mary Mawby, Miss Kathleen Milne, Dr Jean Mitchell, Dr J. Moor, Mrs Alison Murray, (Dr Alison Kirk,) Miss Molly Newby (Durham F.P.C.), Dr M. O'Neill, Dr J. Noble, O.B.E., Dr G. Pearson, Mrs Marion Roberts, Dr J.M. Robertson. Mr. G. Romaines, Mrs Dorothy Salmon, Dr B.S. Sarnaik, Miss Beatrix Scott, Dr C.M. Scott, Dr H.J. Shuttleworth, Mr. W. Skee, the late Dr G.C. Slade, Dr E. Staines, Mrs Ida Staley, Mr J. Stephenson, Mrs Eva Sterling, Dr Elizabeth Sutherland, Mrs Ella Tanfield, Dr D. Thomson O.B.E., J.P. Dr Betty Thomson, Dr R.H. Thorp, Mr F. Vasey, Dr L.G. Velangi, Dr C. Waine, Mrs Mary Walls S.R.N.S.C.M., Mrs Elizabeth Whalen, Mr C. White, Mrs Betty Wilsher and Dr S.K. Young.

We are particularly indebted to Mrs Erika Wallis, Chairman of the S.W.D.H.A. and Mr David Ryan, General Manager of the S.W.D.H.A. for the encouragement they have given us and for the secretarial help they have made available. As a result it is a pleasure to record our thanks to Mrs Angela Fleming and Mrs Diane Harrington for their co-operation and to Mrs Jean Hyslop and Mrs Sheila Featherstone who have patiently typed and retyped the script. We are very grateful to Dr R. McManners for designing the cover and illustrating the map of the S.W. Durham Health District and to Mr G.H. Metcalfe M.A. for reading the manuscripts and for his helpful suggestions. We hope that we have thanked everyone who has made a contribution to the book or who has assisted us in one way or another but to anyone whom we may have forgotten inadvertantly we offer our apologies and thanks.

A.J.A.F.
D.T.P.

Preface to Parts I, II and III

In order to understand the present it is necessary to know something of the past, and to this end we have tried to paint as broad a picture as possible of general practice before the National Health Service. In addition we have tried to trace the origins of all the practices in the South West Durham Health Authority, (the "South West Durham" of the title) and to record the development of general practice from that momentous day in July, 1948, to the present time. We are very grateful to the many doctors and their families who have responded to our request for information. There is a common theme in most of their contributions, namely the virtual disappearance of such diseases as pulmonary tuberculosis, diptheria, and poliomyelitis, the discovery of powerful and effective anti-bacterial drugs, the advent of the National Health Service, the establishment of the District General Hospitals, the decline of domicillary midwifery, improved housing for large numbers of the population, and the formation of groups of doctors practising from purpose built premises.

As well as the historical background to the medical services there are contr-butions illustrating the strong bond between general practitioners and their patients, and there are affectionate recollections by the children who grew up in homes in which "The Surgery" was an integral part.

A great deal of information has come our way and in trying to keep the narrative as concise as possible the problem has been what to omit; we can only hope that we have done justice to all the contributions.

A.J.A.F.
D.T.P.

Throughout the text the National Health Service is referred to as the N.H.S., the National Health Insurance Act (of 1911) as the N.H.I. and the South West Durham Health Authority as the S.W.D.H.A.

PART I

General Practice before the National Health Service

by

A.J.A. Ferguson MB.BS F.R.C.G.P.
Retired General Practitioner, Bishop Auckland.

Contents

Chapter I

The Patchwork Quilt

"The past is a foreign country; they do things differently there."
The Go-Between, L.P. Hartley

There was at least one doctor in this part of County Durham as long ago as 1582, when Roger Gifford described as a Doctor of Physick lived in Tunstall House, Wolsingham Park Head. Doubtless there were others but the earliest record that is available of a general practice in the modern understanding of that term, is one started by Dr Andrew Hewitson of Butts House, Stanhope in 1823. It is known that there were practices in and around Bishop Auckland by the mid 19th century and that about the same time practices sprang up in Crook, Willington, Shildon, Sedgefield, Ferryhill and in the surrounding villages.

Except in cases where medical care was provided through the Poor Law, a fee for service was the basis of the financial relationship between patient and doctor. However, as early as 1900 Insurance Companies and Friendly Societies in industrial cities such as Manchester and Birmingham were moving into the market and providing some sort of medical care for about half the working population, and it was this which formed the framework of the National Health Insurance Act (N.H.I.) of 1911. This Act, piloted through Parliament by Lloyd George and which became operative the following year provided medical care for workers between the age of sixteen and sixty five whose income did not exceed £160 per annum, a limit which was raised to £250 in 1919 and to £420 in 1942.

It was a contributory scheme, compulsory for employer, employee, and the state, each providing a share of the cost of the weekly insurance stamp.[1] The Act, however, excluded not only people whose income exceeded £160 per annum (and the subsequent increases), but housewives, children, self-employed persons and those aged over sixty five. Patients who qualified for care under the N.H.I. registered with the doctor of their choice, provided of course that he had agreed to join the scheme; by no means all of them did, at any rate in the first few months of 1912. Initially the British Medical Association (B.M.A.) advised its members to boycott the scheme but later relented when many of the members resigned in order to join the N.H.I.. Sickness, injury, and maternity benefits were financed by the Insurance Companies and Friendly Societies and were paid at the rate of ten shillings per week for the first twenty six weeks of incapacity and five shillings per week thereafter up to the age of seventy when it ceased; maternity benefit was a single payment of thirty shillings. Prescriptions were confined strictly to those remedies included in the National Formulary which was published in 1912, and subsequently amended from time to time. N.H.I. patients

1. *In 1912 the employer paid 3d, the employee 4d and the state 2d per week.*

provided the general practioner with an unspectacular but steady income, irrespective of whether or not the patient sought advice. By 1948, just prior to the introduction of the N.H.S., the fee for each patient on the doctors list or "panel" as it was then known, had risen to 12s. 6d. per year. What the N.H.I. did not provide was hospital care. This was the province of the Poor Law, the voluntary hospitals and the municipal hospitals. However it did provide some, but not all sanatorium care for patients with tuberculosis.[2]

By the 1920's maternity services, unless privately arranged between the expectant mother and doctor were the responsibility of the County Medical Services which provided ante-natal clinics and the services of a midwife at the time of the confinement.

The health services introduced in this century have fostered the belief that as a nation we were the pioneers of this field. The truth is that we lagged some way behind Germany where that formidable statesman Bismark had the foresight to recognise the importance of medical care particularly for industrial workers whose out-put he hoped would soon rival and then surpass that of Great Britain. To this end he introduced a compulsory health insurance scheme in 1883. In the meantime we got by with a characteristic compromise made up of the Poor Law and voluntary contributory schemes fortified by the N.H.I. until they all disappeared with the introduction of the N.H.S. in 1948.

Those who could not afford private medical care and who were excluded from the N.H.I. for one reason or another could obtain the services of a general practitioner through his "Club". For sixpence a week in the 1920's and 1930's the housewife and her children were entitled to consultations in the surgery, home visits, and the appropriate medication which was dispensed at the doctor's surgery. Widows paid as little as 3d. per week. Even allowing for inflation since then it was remarkably good value. By the end of the 1939/45 War the weekly contributions had risen to 1s. 3d. It was a laudible attempt to provide a medical service in what had been an area of high unemployment and low income.

The contributions were collected in one of two ways. The general practitioner employed a collector who was sometimes his dispenser or perhaps someone specially appointed for the task. They made door to door collections at weekly or fortnightly intervals. In the coal mines around Bishop Auckland owned by Bolckow Vaughan, the club contributions for the miners dependants were deducted at source and paid directly to the colliery doctor. Some people were so poor that they were unable to afford even the club contributions and their medical care was provided by the Parish Doctor as part of his duties as Medical Officer to the Poor Law. These families often received help from the Parochial Church Council's Sick and Poor Fund. With the achievement of something like full employment in the years immediately prior to the last War, and following it, there was scarcely anyone "on the parish" by the time the N.H.S. was introduced in 1948.

2. *There was an increase in the sickness benefit paid to sanatorium cases.*

The General Practitioner

General practitioners worked either on their own or with the help of an assistant or in partnership with another doctor; it was unusual for partnerships to be any larger than two. They worked in accommodation collectively referred to as "The Surgery" which was usually an integral part of their house or built onto it or within its grounds. Surgery accommodation which included the consulting rooms and waiting room varied from practice to practice. Generally speaking it was quite spacious and in some cases represented a considerable sacrifice by the doctor's wife who, in surrendering two rooms of her home often lost accommodation which she would have liked to have for herself and her family. Adjacent to or sometimes within the waiting room was the dispensary which served not only its eponymous duties but was also the nerve centre of the practice. Here a single hand dispenser presided over the order of merit for consultation with the doctor, dispensed bottles of medicine, filled cardboard boxes with tablets and ointments, answered the telephone, made out the visiting lists for the day, kept the accounts, and brewed the tea!

In order to cope with those patients who lived in villages some distance from the main surgery many practices had one and occasionally two branch surgeries. Usually these were more sparsely furnished and equipped than the main surgery and although they may have been frowned upon by those favouring centralised general practice it has to be remembered that in those days transport was a problem and by no means everyone could get to the main surgery as easily as they can do today. As a result the branch surgery served a useful purpose and was understandably popular with the local community — just ask any doctor who closed one!

Where no branch surgery existed and the patients lived some distance from the main surgery there were Call-houses where messages could be left asking the doctor to make a home visit. These Call houses were visited by the doctor only on certain days of the week. A message could always be delivered to the main surgery somehow or other in the event of an emergency but it was amazing how strictly the patients observed the un-written rule and waited for "visiting day". The people who ran the Call houses gave wonderfully loyal and responsible service to the general practitioners until the telephone and motor car made them redundant.

The following description by Dr Janet Alstead (formerly Dr Janet Pope), who was an assistant in a practice in Spennymoor from 1937 to 1943 reveals the scope and responsibility of general practitioners in those times, the long hours of work and in this instance, the basic accommodation.

"The surgery premises were spacious and could have been well adapted to group practice standards as we know them in recent years. Unfortunately most of the rooms remained empty, opening into a large square hall which would have made an excellent waiting room. For some unknown reason instead of using this available space the surgery premises were confined to what was virtually a little dispensing pharmacy. The patient entered a very small waiting room directly from the road with six or eight chairs around the wall. My employer, myself and a dispenser stood behind a counter handing over the appropriate bottles or pills. We had a washbasin and a cold water tap which was in constant use to make up bottles of medicine. Occasionally the patient, having called out his symptoms, was invited to step behind the counter and was escorted to a remote cold room with an examination couch. They imagined that there must be something seriously wrong if they were invited to undress instead of being sent off with a bottle which they had really come for! As my employer became increasingly deaf the lack of privacy in shouting out embarassing complaints in the hearing of others made it imperative to develop a suitable consulting room — much to my delight. I took great pleasure in furnishing this and getting up-to-date equipment. We now had privacy, more time, and facilities for blood counts and microscopic examinations. The dispenser left for war service and was not replaced, and this meant a considerable amount of extra work for me. The evenings were occupied making up large stocks of stomach mixtures and cough mixtures in order to be sure that "the shop" was stocked for the next days onslaught. Any spare time was spent in making up the bills.

We had three surgery sessions a day, 9 to 11 in the morning, 2 to 3 in the afternoon and 6 to 9 in the evening, Saturdays included, and 2 to 3 on Sunday afternoons which I did not like one bit! The home visits were very much more numerous than present day because of lack of effective medicines and because patients were being looked after at home instead of in hospital. It was often necessary to keep an eye on their progress each day or perhaps every other day. The result was fifteen to thirty home visits daily. Private patients such as teachers and businessmen paid about half-a-crown a visit at the surgery and 5s. for a home visit, medicines included.

I can recall many measles, whooping cough and chicken pox epidemics with very ill children, a few polio cases and certainly diptheria, but mostly chest complaints; bronchitis and emphysema and of course tuberculosis. The miners suffered many accidents and fractures which were attended to at Durham County Hospital which was mostly staffed by general practitioners. Domiciliary midwifery was a very exacting and worrying experience. Most of the cases were confined at home and this meant a lot of night work. I can remember many difficult forcep deliveries at home, mercifully without loss of life, either foetal or maternal. I have been back twenty five to thirty years later to wedding ceremonies of some of these difficult cases at the request of the grateful mother!"

Visiting the sick

The tradition of visiting patients in their own home is probably stronger in the North-East than elsewhere in the country although ease of access to health centres and effective treatment has reduced its frequency.

When general practice first became an organised form of medical care in the mid and late 19th century the horse or horse and trap provided transport for the doctor. From lower and upper Weardale the doctors travelled

Visiting the Sick

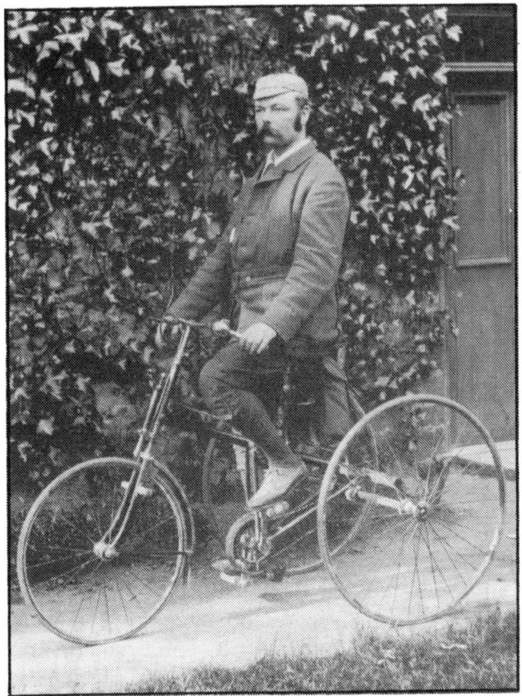

Dr Mark Wardle on his tricycle, about 1900

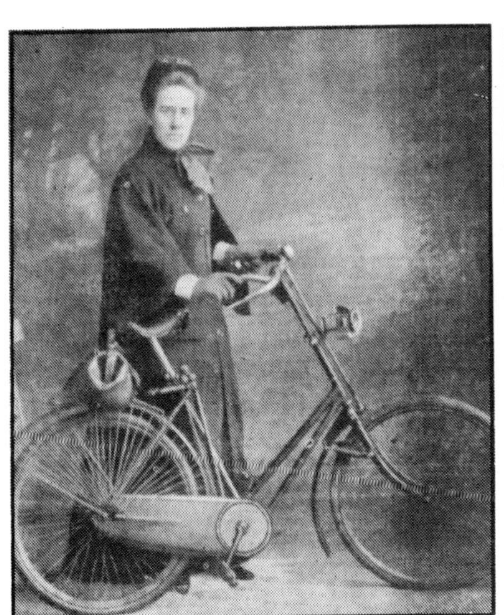

Nurse Violet Wood, about 1925.

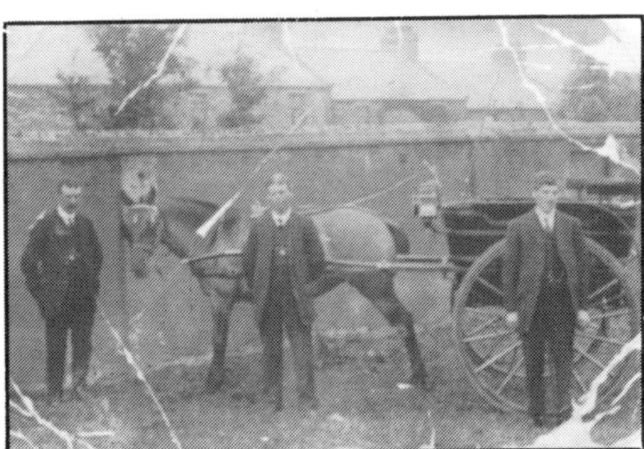

Dr Thorpe's pony and trap with three members of the Duff family of Eldon, about 1900.

each day to the outlying villages on horseback returning to their practice headquarters at night. The doctor wore a wide flared riding coat, the skirt of which was sufficient to cover his legs and most of the horse's back. In the lining of the skirt were pockets in which various medical items were carried, one such was a leather case about the size and shape of a standard book. When opened each side contained six small bottles of concentrated tinctures and in the middle, in the spine of the case, was a small measuring glass. The bottles would contain tinctures of such drugs as opium, belladonna and colchicum, so that a few drops diluted in water would make a single dose for someone requiring quick relief from painful symptoms.

A horse and trap was used whenever and wherever roads permitted, at that time probably only in or around the main towns and larger villages. One well known practitioner, Dr G.W. Ellis of Bishop Auckland, was killed when his pony and trap was involved in an accident in Newgate Street, in 1902. Motorcycles and motor cars replaced the horse just before the Great War although some people can still remember Dr Mark Wardle doing his rounds on a tricycle which disappeared the day he died, never to be seen again. Some of the motorcycles and cars are well remembered, for example the vertically tanked motorcycle of Dr Reubens, sometime assistant to Dr R.W. Smeddle of Shildon, and the bull-nosed Morris of Dr T.E. Ferguson of Bishop Auckland. Also remembered are the chauffeur driven cars of Dr P.V. Anderson of Shildon, Dr Fenwick Lishman of Crook and Dr D.B. Cama of Bishop Auckland.

The arrival of the farm tractor had a profound effect on general practice as Dr Donald Thompson recalls:

"To understand how I feel towards the invention of the farm tractor one must first of all know the general picture of farming in the upper half of Weardale. The valley is fairly shallow with a road running along its lowest line. Along either side of the road the ground rises steadily up to the fells where only heather grows. The area between the road and the edge of the fells is one of green fields used to produce hay for winter feeding of sheep, which is the commonest type of farming. The curious feature is that the farmsteads were originally built not by the roadside but up at the upper edge of the green fields area. The reason for this is very simple. The heaviest load the farm horses had to draw were loads of manure to spread on the fields, the lightest loads were the dry loose hay harvested in the late summer. Heavy loads were led downhill and the lightest loads drawn uphill. The fields were all separated by fences or stone walls or both. The journey from the road to the farm therefore was across these fields and through several gates and these gates had to be left closed. I often had the impression that this was a sacred ritual from centuries past. Through the gates were the soft and muddy tracks left by horse drawn carts. In the 1930's visiting any of these farms was a messy, bumpy and time consuming business, the tracks were nicknamed "The General Practitioners' Obstacle Course"! Although I did not realise it then help was already on the way, the farm tractor had just been invented but was not in general use. After 1945 the use of the farm tractor spread very rapidly through the dales, every farm had one and the bigger farm had two or three. The farm tractor had an immediate and profound effect. The farmer was introduced to the internal combustion engine, which he could take on the road only if he had a driving licence. He quickly got a driving licence and from there quickly got himself a motor car, usually a large one; you cannot carry four pigs in a "Mini"! Now the farmer himself had to travel the obstacle course and close the sacred gates. He quite obviously did not enjoy this experience and gates began to disappear, to be replaced by cattle grids and fencing. The soft muddy tracks were replaced with hard core making it much firmer, and eventually the roads to the farms were smooth tarmac surfaces with no gates. One farm stands out in my memory. It had no fewer than fourteen gates, each gate had to be opened and closed on the way up and again on the way down. I still visit that farm and what a pleasure it is on a lovely summer day to drive up that beautiful hillside on a good tarmac surface and not have to open or close one single gate! I know for certain that the Weardale farmer thanks God for the invention of the farm tractor but there is one former country doctor who does so even more fervently than any farmer!"

The General Practitioner and the Coal Mining Industry

General practitioners in the mining towns and villages before the decline of the coal industry remember those days with affection tinged with sadness. Dr Jean Mitchel assistant to Dr R.A. Brown at Willington, vividly recalls the dangers inherent in the mining industry:-

"Dr Brown was the official colliery surgeon and despite the wonderfully efficient first aid teams every man injured in the colliery had to be seen by the doctor and his injuries entered in an official accident book. Consequently the sound of the colliery ambulance coming down the cul-de-sac to the surgery was a very frequent occurence. One day I had just driven past the Gas House on the colliery road when the whole thing blew up scattering tiles and bricks in all directions. I got out of my car to see if I was needed when four men came running from the nearby colliery rows and a first aid team came pelting down from the colliery and there was a crowd of willing helpers to get the men from under the ruins. No one was killed on that occasion and the injured men recovered, but during my time in Willington four men were killed by falls of stone underground, and on each occasion my car was flagged down and I had to drive up to the colliery mortuary and wait in sad silence until the body was brought up for me to examine. But Willington has a great sense of continuity and self sufficiency; they were such a friendly, closely knit, courageous lot of people. I loved working with them."

Dr John Corrigan of Spennymoor describes his experiences as a colliery doctor:

"If you did not have a reason to go underground in a coal mine over forty years ago as I did, you could not have the faintest conception of the working conditions the miners edured, or of the dangers they faced, although it is true that improvements were introduced at or about that time. One of the most important was the method of supporting the roof and the method of proceeding from the bottom of the mine shaft to the coal face.

On my first trip underground I formed the opinion, which I still maintain, that miners are a breed apart. They struggled away in the bowels of the earth in places where most people would be frightened out of their lives. The darkness, the dust and the claustrophobic atmosphere made life very difficult. The prevalence of chest conditions such as chronic bronchitis and emphysema amongst the miners was not surprising. The method of ventilation resulted in the situation where if the workman was facing in the direction of the oncoming draught of air, his face and hands were showered with a cloud of coal dust as also was his clothing. After the shift a good hot bath was obligatory. At this time there were no such things as pit head baths, the miners still used their old tin bath in front of the fire at home. Miners have always been very fastidious about cleanliness and hygiene and it is greatly to their credit that they always kept up such high standards."

Dr Jack Moor of Crook remembers the 1930's in a mining community.

"Dr Fenwick Lishman and I were the accident doctors for the Colliery. There were all too many fractured spines and severe head injuries. Most were treated at hospital after X-ray, but some returned to us to do what we could with the help of the District Nurses. I became an Assistant Honorary Surgeon at Durham County Hospital after three or four years. Mr J.K. Stanger, an old friend, was Orthopaedic Consultant and Mr J. Hamilton Barclay was Surgical Consultant; they were absolutely invaluable both to me and my patients."

Social Conditions

Most of the miners lived close to their work and their houses were within the shadow of the pit heap and all the unsightly trappings of the coal mining industry. Many of their homes and the homes of other workers had no bathroom or water closet. There was an earth closet across the yard, and in the centre of the yard stood a single cold water tap shared by one or two other households; such conditions prevailed as late as the mid fifties. However, once across the scoured stone doorstep the visitor was in a different world; inside all was as bright and cheerful as it could be made.

The kitchen was the hub of family life. Here the housewife cooked, baked, and washed the dishes and the family bathed in a portable tin tub. There was a large kitchen range which was blackleaded each week. The metal levers and the brass knobs which operated the oven door and the fire draught to the set pot where the water was heated shone brightly.

Monday was the traditional washing day and the clothes were taken out to the poss tub which stood in the yard. These were barrel-like structures filled with hot soapy water. The clothing was pounded either by a single or double poss-stick. Using the latter involved some skill, alternate strokes had to be perfectly timed, otherwise one of the operators received a sharp blow on the shin from the tub. Ironing the clothes was done with a flat iron heated at the kitchen range. If these were "The Good Old Days" they must seem so only in retrospect and no-one can seriously lament their passing.

The miners, who spent their working day below ground, appreciated all that nature could offer above and many were keen gardeners working in their small plots usually some distance from their homes. These were a source not only of flowers, potatoes, cabbages, lettuce and so on but of that Monarch of the Vegetable World, The Prize Leek. They bred racing pigeons and the crees with their fluttering inhabitants were a common sight. There is a splendid quotation in the book "Durham" by Sir Timothy Eden concerning a meeting of the miners of Wheatley Hill Colliery to protest about its threatened closure: "On the same day there was a pigeon race and the pigeons were expected to arrive back from Newcastle at any moment. Just as the orator was in the middle of an impassioned piece of rhetoric, a voice suddenly cried out "Haad thee hand till the "Slate Cock" comes in". The speech ceased immediately and all eyes were upturned to the sky in silent expectation when, like an arrow from a bow, the expected favourite whistled over the heads of the crowd and landed on his ducket. Then the same voice said very deliberately, "There noo, he's landed. Thou can gan on with thee speech"![3]

They bred greyhounds and whippets too, and many were outstanding cricketers and footballers. Jimmy Seed from Whitburn who managed Charlton Athletic in the 1930's and took the London side from the Third Division South into the First Division in successive seasons used to say "If you want a good footballer just go to the top of a pit shaft in County Durham and shout 'Does anyone down there want to play football?,' and up they'll come!"

Care and Treatment

Until well into the 20th century almost all the advances affecting the health of the citizens of Great Britain with the exception of the rapidly expanding field of surgery, were due to public health measures such as vaccination against smallpox and the provision of clean drinking water. The earliest hint of the shape of things to come was the use of arsenical compounds by Ehrlich[4] in 1910 to kill the spirochete causing syphilis by actually attacking it in the patients body. Unhappily like many subsequent anti-bacterial drugs it had unpleasant and sometimes serious side effects. Nevertheless, it was a very significant discovery. There were no further advances in chemotherapy until 1935 when Domagk[5] discovered the first of the sulphonamide drugs, Prontosil, a powerful anti-streptococcal agent. This was followed in the 1940's by the commercial production of Penicillin whose anti-bacterial

3. *"Durham", Sir Timothy Eden. Vol. II, Page 449.*
4. *Paul Ehrlich, German Bacteriologist*
5. *Domagk, German Bacteriologist*

properties had been noted by Sir Alexander Fleming in his laboratory in St. Mary's Hospital, London in 1928. Later other substances were discovered which either killed bacteria in the body or interferred with their multiplication so that the natural defences of the body triumphed over the invaders. The era of antibiotics had dawned and it changed all our lives for the better.

These discoveries were not the result of the introduction of the N.H.S., they were co-incidental, but it did mean that they were available to everyone through the agency of the N.H.S.

The following contributions illustrate what it was like to be a patient and a doctor between the two wars.

From Mr Robert Lewis of Close House, Eldon, Bishop Auckland:

"I was born on 2nd May, 1911, and lived in a terrace house with my parents and brother in Close House, where our doctor was Dr Mason. He was a short, stocky man who spoke with a distinctive Scottish accent. His practice was quite large and widely scattered and every day he did his visiting in a horse drawn trap. He had a surgery every night, except Saturday and Sunday, and this lasted for two or three hours. He was not only a general practitioner, he also did surgical operations such as amputations down the mine when there had been an accident. He also extracted teeth; my mother had her two upper front teeth extracted and I had two molars pulled. There was no "namby pamby" treatment such as cocaine or a painkiller. When I had my teeth drawn I went to the evening surgery and this alone was quite a harrowing experience. There was no receptionist and the waiting room was a bitterly cold place, even in summer, with a bare concrete floor and benches round the walls.

The room always quickly filled with patients and the overflow had to wait outside in the back yard. When you came in, you asked who was last, and you kept that person's face in mind and went into the surgery when he or she came out. The surgery was a cold, narrow room with a gas lamp, lots of bottles, some beakers, a sink and a cold tap. When I got in he asked what was wrong and I told him I had toothache and my mother thought I should have two teeth out. After examining my teeth, and I remember distinctly that his hands were like ice, he took from a drawer what looked to me like a roll-up tool kit, from this he took forceps. He said to me "Put your hands deep in your pockets, don't make a noise and sit still". I will never forget what happened next as long as I live, he put those ice cold forceps on the chosen tooth, pushed them down through the gums, gripped and rocked the tooth and pulled it out with a sort of sucking noise, threw the tooth in the sink and repeated on the other tooth."

Here Mr Lewis remembers the poverty, the diseases and the social conditions prevalent at the time.

"In those days there was a lot of poverty and malnutrition and at school rickets and ringworm were quite common but of course the killers were tuberculosis, diphtheria and scarlet fever. Nobody had WCs or running hot water. In Close House every house had earth closets in the back yard but some streets in Eldon had open middens and the closets were across quite a wide road, a mud road and, I may add, very muddy in wet weather".

Local Authority Clinics

Child Welfare and other local authority clinics such as Ante-natal Clinics were usually held in old houses or halls large enough to be adapted for the purpose. In Bishop Auckland for example these clinics were in Ninefields, a large house on Etherley Lane which has since been demolished. Their origin is interesting; individual Medical Officers of Health in provincial cities and towns had achieved striking reductions in infant mortality by the introduction of Child Welfare Clinics, the principle being that of reaching the individual mother and teaching her how to rear her infant. Just as was the case with our N.H.I. we were not the originators, the credit in this instance going to France where the movement began in 1890 and was known as Goutte de Lait (literally a drop or sip of milk), its purpose being to provide reliable free milk to poor mothers. The earliest English equivalent was started in St. Helens, Lancashire in 1899, and within a few years there were a dozen or more in the provinces. There was, however, one branch of health supervision in which we were the pioneers and that was the visiting of the poor and needy in their homes by non-medical personnel. This began in 1862 in Manchester and Salford, when the first members of the movement were women volunteers acting as social reformers. Their visits were a mixture of philanthropy, evangelism and carbolic. By the 1890's the work of these dedicated women was beginning to be recognised by the more progressive Medical Officers of Health, in particular by Dr Samson Moore of Huddersfield. A visit to Huddersfield to see how things were done there became almost a pilgrimage for those concerned with Child Welfare.

Gradually the volunteers were replaced by properly trained professional Health Visitors and they assumed an increasingly important role in the care and supervision of infants, children and the elderly. Today, no Primary Health Care Team is complete without the Health Visitor.

Ante-natal Clinics provided the regular supervision of the expectant mother which is so essential in detecting conditions harmful to her and her unborn child. It was here that she was looked after by the midwife, who would attend her during her confinement at home, where the vast majority of confinements took place. The attending midwife was entitled to seek the help of the patient's doctor for whatever she judged necessary, which might include an obstetrical procedure such as a forceps delivery. Occasionally, where the nature of the emergency was such that a Consultant Obstetrician's expertise was required and the distance to hospital far enough to endanger the patient's life, the Obstetric Flying Squad inaugurated by Professor Farquhar Murray[6] and based in Newcastle-upon-Tyne could be brought speedily to the bedside.

6. *E. Farquhar Murray sometime Professor of Obstetrics and Gynaecology, University of Durham.*

The following description by Mr S. McGreevy, of Shildon, is a typical example of the obstetrical and child welfare services existing in the thirties:

"At that time (1930) nearly all babies were born at home with the help of midwives and local women, who although not qualified were always called for at childbirth. I was a breech baby and weighed only $2^1/_2$ lbs. My mother took me for sunlight treatment at the Welfare Centre which was at the rear of the Friends Meeting House on Byerley Road, Shildon where it continued for many years. It was used for weighing babies, distribution of free baby food, orange juice and any necessary advice.

Our midwives were Nurse Haw, Nurse Nelson or "Grannie" Clark. Only in later years could expectant mothers in difficulty go to Hardwick Hall Maternity Home near Sedgefield or Princes Street Maternity Home, Bishop Auckland, both now closed. The local doctors were Dr Widdas, Dr Anderson and Dr Smeddle".

This contribution from Mr F. Vasey, also of Shildon, illustrates the versatility and ingenuity of the practitioner:

"I fractured my left femur one Saturday afternoon in 1920 playing for Shildon at home in the North Eastern League. I have a vivid memory of Dr Smeddle and the equipment he used. No fancy Thomas splint, no plaster cast! The splints were adjuster lengths of wood normally used to enlarge the area of a quilting or "proddie" mat frame. The traction was a flat iron tied with a length of string to my big toe and allowed to dangle over the end of the wooden settle. Incidentally, it turned out to be a perfect set!"

The District Nursing Services

District Nursing began in Liverpool in 1859 under the direction of Dr William Rathbone. Later the Queen's Nursing Institute, founded in 1887, took up the cause of District Nursing and provided almost all the nurses attending the sick in their homes. They were all State Registered and specially trained for the task. One such was Nurse Violet Wood of Bishop Auckland, a well-known figure riding around the town on her bicycle, her uniform billowing in the wind, and accompanied by a small dog, variously identified as being a Chihuahua, a Pekinese or a Yorkshire Terrier. Whatever the breed, legend has it that she attended a service in Durham Cathedral with the dog concealed under her voluminous cloak. Not being able to follow the service from these dark recesses the dog grew restless and began to bark, whereupon she was asked to leave. It is said that the incident achieved some noteriety in the press. She fell out with the Queen's Nursing Institute, but resolutely continued on her own, raising money for her work by means of Nurse Wood's Violet Day, rather in the manner of a Flag Day, except that in her case the donors were given a violet to pin to their coats. During her professional life-time she did much valuable work for the citizens of Bishop Auckland and particularly for the Durham Miners Association. Everyone who knew her has a clear picture of her in their mind and her name is perpetuated on two hymn book racks which she presented to St Peter's Church in 1938.

Where there were no Queen's Nurses, local Nursing Associations employed the district nurse. These Associations were financed by regular weekly contributions and fund raising events; in Evenwood for instance, in 1933 the weekly contribution was one penny. Sometimes the district nurse was also the midwife, and by 1947 the fee for a home confinement was £2 if the mother was a member of the Association and £3 if she was not.

By the 1930's local authorities were becoming involved, providing both district nurses and midwives. In Bishop Auckland in 1937 qualified midwives employed by Durham County Council replaced the old "handy-women", the unqualified, but by no means despised women who helped general practitioners at home confinements. In the same year the County Council took over the employment of the district nurses from the Bishop Auckland Nursing Association and by 1946 Queen's Nurses represented only 50% of all district nurses. The development of the domiciliary nursing services after the introduction of the N.H.S. is referred to in Part II.

A General Practitioner Looks Back

Dr Jack Moor, in general practice in Crook from 1932 to 1980 apart from the war years in which he served in the Royal Navy, recalls the limited number of really effective drugs available for serious diseases and the professional life style of a doctor before 1939:

"Our dispensary was adequate for its time. There were the usual stock mixtures for coughs and gastro-intestinal upsets and there were asprin tablets, laxative tablets and other symptomatic remedies. Rational treatment, however, was beginning to dawn. Insulin had been discovered in 1922 by Banting and Best[7] but was largely controlled by hospitals. Pernicious Anaemia was treated by raw liver sandwiches — neither palatable nor very effective. Stomach extract was being investigated and fairly soon liver extract injections became available as a result of work by Whipple, Minot and Murphy.[8] We could do simple blood counts in the surgery but scientific control was usually arranged by the hospital. Syphilis was an uncommon disease in Crook but was treated with arsenical compounds and bismuth at V.D. Clinics.

Later in the 1930's the sulphonamides appeared. I treated an elderly gentleman with a carbuncle with my first free sample and was duly amazed and gratified by his rapid recovery. This was probably the first real change in what was strictly "general practitioner treatment" and our lives and our patients lives were never the same again. Penicillin, of course, was still an entry in a laboratory scrap book.

In "quiet" times I did about twenty visits a day, but we had two severe 'flu epidemics in 1932/33 and 1933/34 in which I did forty to sixty visits a day. It was much less severe than the 1918 'flu, but we had a few deaths even in

7. *Canadian Physiologists.*
8. *American Medical Research Workers*

the young. In my opinion it was much more severe than the Asian 'flu of 1957 — and there was no penicillin.

My experience in midwifery had been very limited and I learned a great deal from my senior partner Dr Fenwick Lishman. We did virtually no ante-natal examinations, patients "booked" with the local midwife and we were called only in cases of difficulty, usually delay in labour, occasionally for haemorrhage both before and after the birth of the baby and for cases where stitches were required. Our death rate was surprisingly small which I attribute to a strict aseptic and antiseptic technique. If called by the mid-wives we were paid small but welcome fees by the County Council. The more serious cases were admitted to the Princess Mary Maternity Hospital at Newcastle, and if we were in difficulty Professor Farquhar Murray would willingly come out to Crook to help us, although blood transfusion was not available to us at this time.

My partner Dr Fenwick Lishman was part-time Medical Officer at Helmington Row Isolation Hospital. There were two large wards for scarlet fever and diphtheria and two smaller wards for terminal tuberculosis and other infections, usually meningitis. Here I was able to do tracheotomies and lumbar punctures, these techniques were very useful at sea during the war — but that is another story. Of the killer diseases of the 1930's diphtheria was the worst, but in due course much reduced by mass immunisation in co-operation with the County Medical Officer and his staff. Scarlet fever could be surprisingly severe in this period but later became an almost trivial complaint possibly due to sulphonamides and improved nutrition and hygiene; meningitis at last became treatable with sulphonamides. Pulmonary tuberculosis both in hospital and in the practice was a very tragic illness, almost always fatal, and affecting mostly the younger patients and those of Irish origin. Infantile diarrhoea of a serious type was less common than I had expected and this applied also to lobar pneumonia, "The Captain of the Men of Death".

Two diseases which were surprisingly infrequent and rapidly becoming almost rare by the mid thirties but which we had been led to expect to see in large numbers when we were at medical school were children with rickets and cases of Weardale goitre, the latter being a swelling of the thyroid gland which is situated in the neck. It was a condition with strong family connections which gradually died out due, I think, to the coming of the "Heatherbell" and other Weardale bus services and the consequent cessation of in-breeding.

Rickets, a condition leading to skeletal deformities, was gradually disappearing because Vitamin D, in the form of cod liver oil, was available at the Child Welfare Clinics, where parents were also advised to encourage their children to drink milk — a rich source of calcium. In the larger cities, the gradual clearance of Victorian slums, which had denied children living in them the sunlight so essential to the utilisation of Vitamin D in the body, was another important factor in the eradication of rickets, which in the United Kingdom was essentially a disease of poverty.

Mention of coronary thrombosis must be made as a very infrequent cause of death in the 30 - 60 age groups. Most of those who died relatively young died of pulmonary tuberculosis, which was rife, and the infectious fevers. Many of the 'missing generation' were killed during the 1914/18 war. I can still remember as a young boy seeing page upon page of casualties in the newspapers. Those in these age groups could not die of coronary thrombosis; they had already died".

The Dispensers

Every general practice had a dispenser. They were by no means merely mixers of medicaments. Their duties might include book-keeping, collecting "Club" contributions, some secretarial tasks and driving the doctor on his rounds. Perhaps their most important contribution was their encyclopaedic knowledge of the patient's medical and family histories, their virtues and (occasionally) their vices, and the wise counsel they gave to fledgeling general practitioners.

Amongst this group of versatile men and women were Joe Murphy with Dr Smeddle and later Dr P.V. Anderson's practice, William Harrison followed by Edward Goodfellow and his wife Monnie with Dr Fenwick Lishman's practice and, although she did not drive, Mrs Whalen with Dr Ferguson's practice. They played a vital part in the day to day management of the practices. In a word the dispensers were indispensable.

Some Personal Recollections

Life in a general practitioner's house was certainly different from any other. The disturbances caused by messages coming in over the telephone or at the door were all part of the daily (and sometimes nightly) routine.

The very nature of the general practitioner's work meant that family outings were not quite so frequent as those of many of their friends, but there were compensations. The doctor's children sometimes accompanied him on his visiting rounds especially during the long summer holiday. In this way they got an insight into the life of a general practitioner and, who knows?, it may have inspired one or two of them to follow in father's footsteps. Another treat was to be allowed into the dispensary where there was a display of stock bottles containing cough mixtures, stomach mixtures, ointments, tablets, tinctures and syrups — all bearing abbreviated Latin names. There was a mystique about it which is quite lacking in today's prepackaged products. Modern medicines require a precise dose and the 5 ml. spoon has replaced the time honoured but inaccurate measure of household teaspoons, desert spoons and tablespoons. Also banished to the realms of pharmaceutical history are grains and ounces, now replaced by milligrammes and grammes. Gone too are those esoteric symbols and abbreviations which baffled the layman but which told the dispenser the quantity required and how frequently the dose was to be taken. To be allowed into the dispensary and watch the dispenser at work was more than just a childhood treat, it was akin to an initiation ceremony — a feeling of belonging to the practice.

General practice was very much a family affair in which no-one played a more important rôle than the doctor's wife. Housewife, mother, out of hours telephonist and receptionist, comforter of the anxious relative and ministering angel to her husband, she was and indeed still is, the un-sung heroine of general practice.

When the children grew up they could be quite useful to father as Mrs Dorothy Salmon, daughter of Dr Fenwick Lishman remembers:

"My early memories are of filling medicine bottles with stock mixtures made up by my father in the Witton-le-Wear Call House. I was deputed to go down the yard with an enormous jug which had to be filled with water and then lugged back. Possibly before the war general practitioners helped each other more. I can remember my father doing another doctor's surgeries for which he received a gramophone. In all the years my father and Dr Moore were in partnership it was always "Dr Lishman" and "Dr Moor". Shades of Dr Finlay's Casebook!".

From Dr Maryan Huntridge (younger daughter of Dr W. Anderson) come these amusing vignettes.

"Infusion of gentian root was thought to stimulate the appetite and was also used as a general tonic. It was made up into either acid or alkaline mixtures and labelled in that shorthand Latin so beloved by the profession, Mist Gent Acid, and Mist Gent Alk. For years one doctor's small daughter thought that these mixtures were for men only!"

"In the mining areas where death was thought to be attributable to silicosis, a pathologist would come from Newcastle to carry out the mandatory post mortem examination. It was customary for the pathologist to be invited back to the doctor's house for lunch. On one such occasion he placed a specimen jar on the lunch table and spoke enthusiastically about its contents. Mother was quite horrified until it transpired that the jar contained plums and was a gift from the pathologist's wife!".

From Professor J.R. Anderson (son of Dr W. Anderson):

"Times were hard in the 1920's and 1930's and there were many acts of kindness by general practitioners to poor patients, especially those with chronic disease. At Christmas time it was not uncommon for the 8 fluid ounce bottle of cough medicine to be magically transformed into 8 fluid ounces of whisky and labelled 'Spiritus Fermenti'!"

There were and indeed still are many lighter moments in general practice, but the difference in those days was that many of them involved the doctor's family too. Before public telephone kiosks became so widespread and telephones in homes so common nearly all the requests for night visits were made by a relative or neighbour coming to the doctors house. The sound of the dreaded night bell woke everyone and a sleepy and sometimes rather cross doctor would put his head out of a convenient window near to, or overlooking the front door. From here he would ask the caller questions about the nature of the trouble and, most importantly, the patients address because some messengers had the disconcerting habit of disappearing into the darkness having unburdened themselves of the patient's symptoms, but not the address. In some doctors houses a speaking tube linked the recumbent doctor with the patient and it was said that the appropriate remedy for the complaint, in the shape of tablets of course, sometimes found their way down the same tube!

Mrs Betty Wilsher (elder daughter of Dr W. Anderson) remembers an occasion in the 1930's when the nocturnal caller was a patient known to suffer from a mental illness. "Doctor", he shouted in the direction of the window above, "I cannot get any sleep. They're sending out electric currents from the Hall". "Which side of the bed is your wife sleeping on, on the one next to the Hall"? asked the doctor. "No", replied the patient "she is on the inside". "Well," said the doctor, "just get her to change places with you. They aren't after her and she will absorb the waves and they won't harm her". "Thanks very much doctor, that's grand", replied the patient and quite content he returned to his home. Appropriate action was taken the following morning.

Chapter II

The Making of the National Health Service

The Dawson Report of 1920[8*] suggested the amalgamation of general practice, hospital and public health services under a single health authority and the establishment of primary health centres to be staffed by general practitioners and secondary health centres based on hospitals, rather after the manner of the Casualty Clearing Stations and the Field Hospitals of the Great War. The scheme was to be available to everyone although there was no mention of how it was to be financed. For some reason it failed to capture the imagination of the politicians or the public. Perhaps the former were too preoccupied with the problems of post war Europe, perhaps the latter detected an all too familiar military ring about it, which was precisely what they wanted to forget. Whatever the reason no action was taken and the subject of a comprehensive medical service lay undisturbed until the B.M.A. published its own plan in 1929 under the title "A General Medical Service for the Nation".[9] The report stated four basic principles:

1. *That the system of medical service should be directed to the achievement of positive health and the prevention of disease, no less than to the relief of sickness.*
2. *That there should be provided for each individual a family doctor of his own choice.*
3. *That consultants and specialist laboratory services and all necessary auxiliary services, together with institutional provision when required, should be available for the individual patient through the agency of the family doctor.*
4. *That the several parts of the complete Medical Service should be closely coordinated and developed by the application of a planned N.H.S.*

By 1934 the Labour Party was committed to a free Health Service and they emphasised this at their Party Conference in 1943 when they declared their intention of introducing a whole-time salaried National Health Service if they were elected to form the Government after the war. Nevertheless it is important to recognise the B.M.A.'s foresight and initiative in 1929, not least because the general public often misunderstood the doctor's attitude prior to the introduction of the N.H.S. The difference of opinion was not about *whether* it should be done, but *how* it should be done.

Just how such a scheme was to be financed was rather vague. The economic depression was approaching its lowest point in 1929 and perhaps the B.M.A. like Mr Micawber was waiting for something to turn up. When

8* *Named after Lord Dawson of Penn, a distinguished Physician and Chairman of the Consultative Council on Medical and Allied Services.*

9. *"History of the B.M.A." Vol. II, E. Gray Turner and F.M. Sutherland.*

eventually the depression gave way to almost full employment, mainly due to rearmament just prior to the outbreak of war in 1939, it was too late in the day to be thinking of a comprehensive health service; the Government was preoccupied in preparing the nation to meet the growing threat of Nazi Germany. However, the B.M.A. aware that there would be radical changes in medical practice in Britain after the war, set up a Medical Planning Commission in 1940.

The report published in 1942 was a bold and imaginative document. Paradoxically it made a number of recommendations which when taken up by the wartime coalition Government in its White Paper of 1944 and again in the N.H.S. Bill of 1946 were resolutely opposed by the rank and file members of the B.M.A. itself. Among these recommendations were that general practitioners should be encouraged to group together and work in health centres under the control of regional authorities and that they should be remunerated partly by basic salary and partly by capitation fees. The hospitals were to be administered by the same regional authorities and the consultants offered either full-time or part-time contracts.

Shortly after the Medical Planning Commission's report was published the Government set up an Inter-Departmental Committee on Social Insurance and Allied Services.

The Chairman was Sir William Beveridge and the Committee's deliberations published in December, 1942 were forever afterwards known as the Beveridge Report. The population, encouraged by the recent victory at El Alamein, seized upon the Beveridge Report as the harbinger of A Brave New World which they felt sure would be theirs once the war was over, and as a result it was an instant best seller. Briefly the scheme was to insure the whole Nation against illness, injury, and unemployment and to provide a retirement pension. The necessary funding was to be provided by individual citizens, employers and the Government.[10]

The report assumed, without going into details that "A comprehensive N.H.S. will ensure that for every citizen there is available whatever medical treatment he requires in whatever form he requires it, domiciliary or institutional, general, specialist, or consultant, and will ensure also the provision of dental, opthalmic and surgical appliances, nursing and midwifery and rehabilitation after accidents".[11] Beveridge was not universally popular and many thought that he exceeded the bounds of Civil Service etiquette by personally seeking support for the report amongst Liberal and Socialist members of Parliament. "On the day when the results of the 1945 General Elections were being declared the British Medical Association was holding its Annual Representative Meeting in the Great Hall in Tavistock Square, the BMA Headquarters. Debates were interrupted with the latest Election bulletins, and when the news came through that Sir William Beveridge, Liberal M.P. for Berwick, had been defeated, some delegates broke into a

10. *"History of the B.M.A." Vol. II, E. Grey Turner and F.M. Sutherland*
11. *Ibid.*

cheer which the British Medical Journal preferred later to dismiss as a gasp of astonishment."[12]

Nevertheless in 1942, the Beveridge Report not only caught the imagination of the people but of the politicians too and the Minister of Health, Mr. Ernest Brown, a National Liberal, began a series of discussions with the B.M.A., none of which could be described as fruitful. The Minister put forward the idea of general practitioners being in contract with a Central Medical Board and the local authority owning the health centres in which they would be expected to work. The profession saw this as a service to which it was strongly opposed i.e. a state salaried service under local authorities. The discussions, which were not binding on either side ground to a halt.

Mr Henry Willink, a Conservative M.P. replaced Mr Brown as Minister of Health and shortly aftrwards the Government published a White Paper on a proposed N.H.S.

The 1944 White Paper

As far as general practice was concerned the basis of the proposed Health Service was still to be a whole-time salaried service in health centres owned by local authorities, to which the B.M.A. remained resolutely opposed. Individual local authorities saw their powers being erroded by being made to collaborate with neighbouring local authorities to provide health centres. The voluntary hospitals, although aware of their declining finances, and their need for some sort of state funding in the future, feared for their independence and as a result they too were opposed to the proposals. Lastly those who argued for a radical health service such as the Socialist Medical Association, the Fabian Medical Services Group and burgeoning socialist medico-politicians such as Dr Somerville Hastings and Dr Edith Summerskill regarded the proposals as a compromise. Henry Willink, however, was more flexible than his predecessor and entered into discussions with a newly formed B.M.A. Committee[13] over such vexed questions as the general practitioners loss of right to sell their practices and other sensitive problems such as general practitioners working in local authority health centres. From these discussions stemmed a pamphlet published by the B.M.A. which took the form of questions to, and answers by the Minister in which he tried to allay the professions' worst fears.

Aneurin Bevan erupted in anger claiming that it was unconstitutional for a Minister to discuss proposals with an outside body before reporting them to Parliament, and the B.M.A. got its first taste of things to come. Henry Willink tried hard to please all sides and in the end pleased none. Perhaps it was a relief to the Government that attention to the White Paper was diverted by the signs of approaching victory in Europe. In the event there were to be no further discussions until after the general election called for July, 1945 when, in one of the greatest political upsets of modern times the Labour Party was elected with a huge majority.

12. *"Aneurin Bevan. 1945-1960", Michael Foot*
13. *Dr. P.V. Anderson of Shildon was a member of this Committee.*

Aneurin Bevan and the National Health Service

Clement Atlee, the new Prime Minister appointed Aneurin Bevan as Minister of Health and Housing. Thus by a strange coincidence, at the two most critical occasions in its history, the medical profession was to find itself faced by two Welshmen, Lloyd George with the National Health Insurance Bill in 1911, and Aneurin Bevan with the National Health Service Bill in 1946. Both men were great social reformers and both were capable of stirring oratory.

Bevan had not previously held political office nor was he likely to have done so in a coalition government led by Winston Churchill with whom he had had some bitter exchanges over the conduct of the war and who had once described him as "that squalid nuisance". As far as the general public was concerned he burst upon the political scene with a reputation of being something of a rebel, and a left wing rebel at that.

Given the medical profession's deeply entrenched conservatism and his political reputation the two were on a collision course from the start, but he was by no means the bogyman he was made out to be in some sections of the press.

He was very determined, frequently charming, and occasionally abrasive. In addition he had a penchant for making provocative speeches. He spoke with a lilting Welsh accent and a slight stammer which many people thought he used to good effect. In this way he kept his supporters waiting eagerly for the dénoument so that when it eventually arrived its effect was heightened by anticipation.

He was always elegantly dressed and he was fond of the occasional glass of champagne; not for nothing was he known as the Bolinger Bolshevik. He worked extremely hard at his brief, preferring to answer questions himself rather than rely on his Civil Servants. Everyone who came into contact with him, both supporters and opponents, was amazed at his detailed knowledge of medical practice in every aspect. All this was achieved at the cost of hard work and it is said that he brought a caseful of documents home every night and worked on them in a small bedroom at the top of his house. One night after working away for hours he called to his wife[14] to bring up a second batch of papers. "No" she replied. "One you may have but taking two to bed is immoral!".

He had a lively and occasionally mischevious sense of humour. Once when he was discussing the Maternity Service with Eardley Holland then President of the Royal College of Obstetricians and Gynaecologists, Holland said to him "You see Minister, this is a matter of great importance to me for I am responsible for all the pregnant women in the Country". "You're boasting!" interrupted Bevan.[15]

14. *Jenny Lee, Labour M.P. for Cannock, later Baroness Lee of Asheridge.*
15. *"Aneurin Bevan, 1945-1960", Michael Foot*

The architects of the National Health Service

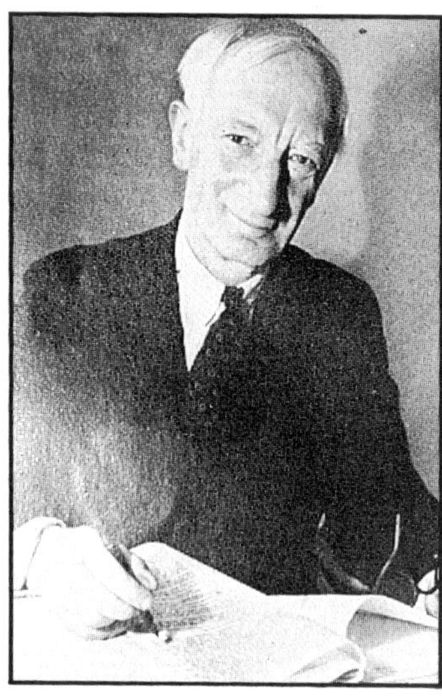

Sir William Beveridge of the famous Beveridge Report.

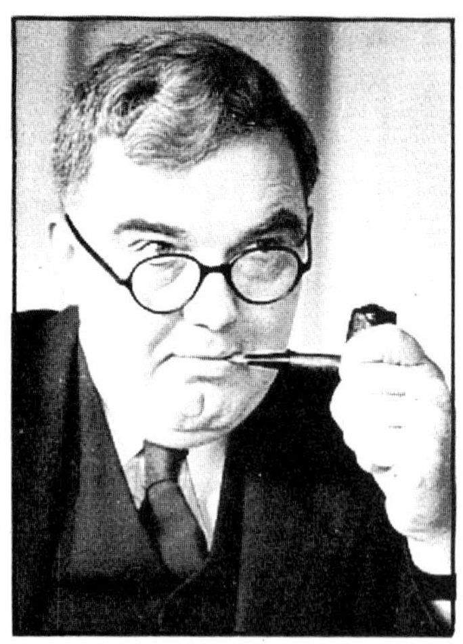

Dr Charles Hill, Secretary, B.M.A.

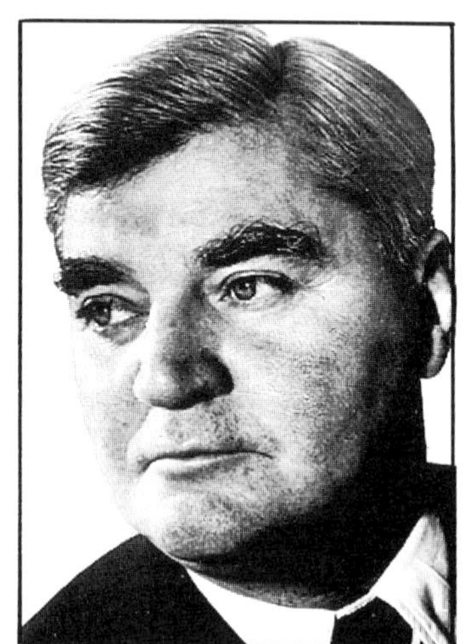

Aneurin Bevan, Minister of Health 1945-51.

It was going to need all his hard work, patience (of which he was rather short sometimes) and certainly all his political skill to win over this conservative profession whose main objection was not to the spirit of the Bill but to its terms of service. Not for them a whole-time salaried service, nor life in health centres owned by local authorities, nor the dictates of faceless mandarins in the Ministry of Health.

The battle was now joined between the standard bearer of the profession, the B.M.A., and the Government as represented by the Minister of Health, Aneurin Bevan. By way of support in Parliament the doctors could count upon the Conservative Party. Outside Parliament the effect of the Labour Party landslide of 1945 was such that many Conservative voters clearly regarded the doctors' stand against Bevan as the last bastion between themselves and the tumbrils waiting to take them to the guillotine. As a result this beleagured group added their support to that of the Tory Press.

To understand the doctors' antipathy to any form of state controlled medical practice it has to be remembered that they had looked after the sick without interference from any quarter until the advent of the N.H.I. in 1912. Its long history of autonomy, its code of conduct, ethics and etiquette made it a much respected profession. The profession was proud of its reputation and not without justification. But over and above all that was the threat to that precious but intangible asset, clinical freedom. A state service it was said would compel obedience to a new master and doctors would no longer be answerable to their patients and their peers. It was not beyond the bounds of possibility, they thought, that these faceless mandarins in the Ministry would dictate how an illness should be treated.

It was against this background that the long and sometimes turbulent negotiations between Bevan and the B.M.A. began.

From the outset there was instant recognition of Bevan's ability and also of his authoritarian attitude which was to antagonise the doctors on occasions. Both are admirably captured in this description of him by Lord Hill in his autobiography.[16]

"We were to find in Aneurin Bevan a formidable negotiator — charming and sympathetic at one moment he could be hotly indignant at the next. In a flash he could spot a flaw in an argument without waiting or wanting to wait for a speaker to finish. He would purr or pounce, according to his mood — gaily argumentative in debate, he preferred giving it to taking it — but so do we all. If a suggestion was unacceptable to him he said so at once — never using the comforting formula that the matter would be considered when he really rejected it. I do not remember any occasion on which he said one thing and meant another — this was part of the trouble at certain moments."

16. *"Both Sides of the Hill", Lord Hill of Luton formerly Charles Hill, Secretary of the B.M.A. 1944 - 1950, and war-time "Radio Doctor".*

In March, 1946, Aneurin Bevan presented his N.H.S. Bill to Parliament. For practical purposes Clause I of the Bill stated the main aim:

"It shall be the duty of the Minister of Health to promote the establishment in England and Wales[17] of a comprehensive Health Service designed to secure improvement in the physical and mental health of the people of England and Wales and the prevention, diagnosis and treatment of illness, and for that purpose to provide or secure the effective provision of services in accordance with the following provisions of this Act.

The service so provided shall be free of charge, except where any provision of this Act expressly provides for the making and recovery of charges".

This last sentence was to have dramatic repercussions five years later when Aneurin Bevan, by then Minister of Labour, resigned from the Cabinet as a protest over the introduction of charges for spectacles and dentures and the threat of prescription charges.

The Bill became law in November, 1946. During this period the B.M.A. complained that Bevan had not entered into negotiations with them as had previous Ministers of Health but bearing in mind his reaction to Henry Willink's tentative steps in this direction in 1945 he was not likely to have put into practise as a Minister what he had so vehemently criticised as a back bencher in 1945. Nevertheless it was known that during this time he had taken soundings from certain influential members of the profession including Lord Moran, President of the Royal College of Physicians who was known to be sympathetic to the principles involved in a National Health Service.

Now that it was on the statute book negotiations could begin in earnest because the service was scheduled to start in July, 1948. The main stumbling block as far as the general practitioner services were concerned was undoubtedly the spectre of a full-time salaried service. Bevan's proposal was that doctors' remuneration should be partly by basic salary and partly by capitation fee and it was the basic salary that struck fear into the general practitioners hearts. It was only a step from here, they feared, to a full-time salaried service. Bevan later conceded payment by capitation fee only, although in fairness to him he thought that it was a mistake for the doctors to insist upon this. Indeed remuneration of general practitioners purely by the capitation system proved to be a thorny problem throughout the first two decades of the service. Ironically the basic salary under the guise of the Basic Practice Allowance was the cornerstone of the profession's famous "Doctor's Charter" of 1967; had Bevan been alive then he would have been justified in feeling that his original proposal had been the right one.

The Bill granted the right to doctors who joined the service to continue with private practice if they so wished, although it was anticipated that this would soon disappear with the establishment of a well run N.H.S. The Bill

17. *There was a separate Bill for Scotland.*

also allowed doctors to take up private appointments such as Medical Officers to private industry and to serve on Industrial Injury and War Pension Medical Boards and similar appointments which were not within the remit of the N.H.S.

Doctors were to be in contract with Executive Councils (serving each county or a single large city) and compensation for the loss of the right to sell their practices was agreed to with surprisingly little discord although its payment was delayed for many years.

But the general practitioners remained hesitant and plebiscites carried out by the B.M.A. in 1946, and again early in 1948, showed that the vast majority of doctors disaproved of the Act in its present form — they still feared that a whole-time salaried service could be introduced by a regulation of the Act, if not by Bevan himself then by some future Minister of Health.

To overcome this impasse Bevan introduced an Amendment to the Act making it clear that new Parliamentary Legislation would be necessary before this could happen. Whether or not it was the Government's intention eventually to introduce a full-time salaried service either in this Parliament or in the next, if they were re-elected, is one of the political mysteries of those times, but the B.M.A. can be justifiably proud of its resolute stand and its successful outcome.

The Hospital Service

Michael Foot describes how, in the National Health Service Bill of 1946, "Bevan proposed an expropriation of all hospitals, while leaving the teaching hospitals a separate status, a special control over their endowments and a special method of nomination to their Board of Governors. Here indeed was one of Bevan's crucial decisions, for only by attracting the best and most prestigious medical brains into the service could he hope to make it universal, covering the whole or nearly the whole population. Authority over the hospital system, for both planning and supervision, would then, in Bevan's plan, be delegated to fourteen Regional Boards appointed by the Ministry and through them to Local Management Committees".[18]

The proposal got a hostile reception from the B.M.A. who saw this as a dictatorial move and one which would destroy the proud tradition of the voluntary hospitals. But the doctors working in the voluntary hospitals were only too well aware of the constraints due to inadequate financial resources. In addition by no means all the doctors working in the municipal hospitals were convinced that these were the ideal alternative — standards varied from one local authority to another.

Bevan reasoned that if the salaries were attractive and the work interesting then the best consultants could be tempted away from the teaching centres

18. "Aneurin Bevan, 1945 - 1960", Michael Foot.

and the large city hospitals and he could halt the hitherto uneven distribution of Consultants throughout the country. If they had the added attraction of private beds in the N.H.S. hospitals then that, he argued, would encourage them to work in the hospitals rather than in private nursing homes.

In this way Bevan justified his proposals for allowing private beds in N.H.S. hospitals to his colleagues in the Cabinet and to the zealots of the Labour Party who regarded private patients either inside or outside a hospital as anathema. It is said, however, that when discussing his plans for the consultants with friends privately, he claimed he had "Stuffed their mouths with gold"!

It was clear that from this time on, the majority of the consultants backed by the Royal Colleges were ready to start work in the N.H.S. on the 5th July, 1948, long before the general practitioners were ready. This created some ill feeling between the B.M.A. and the Royal Colleges which was to last well into the life time of the N.H.S. The B.M.A. had always hoped to strengthen their case by presenting a united front. In the meantime there was a perceptible change in the attitude of the general practitioners at the grass roots.

Bevan's amendment to the Act along with the B.M.A's. insistence on remuneration solely by capitation fee certainly had much to do with this change. In addition there was a growing enthusiasm amongst the younger doctors to take up the challenge of being in the vanguard of the worlds first comprehensive medical service.
There was another but much less altruistic reason within the ranks of general practitioners; there was a hint of skulduggery at the grass roots. At local B.M.A. meetings the air was thick with cigarette smoke and duplicity. Some doctors, fearing a repetition of 1912, when loyalty to the B.M.A. cost them dearly, were not going to be left stranded this time and they instructed their "Club" collectors to make sure that the families had completed their N.H.S. registration forms in favour of "The Old Firm". In the meantime the same doctors protested vigorously against the iniquities of the terms of service and supported motions not to disclose by any means whatsoever their intentions of joining the service until permitted to do so by the B.M.A.! Such perfidious behaviour was encouraged by the rumour, perhaps strategically put about, that those who did not join the N.H.S. on the appointed day would forfeit their compensation for the loss of right to sell their practices. In the meantime there was a steady alienation of public opinion. Now that general practitioners had won the assurance that they were not to become full-time salaried servants of the state, that they were to be paid by a method of their own choosing and were to be allowed private practice if they wished, what was it that made them hesitate? The public was growing tired of this seemingly endless rearguard action. It was beginning to look as if the B.M.A's. critics were right in the end; that it paid lip service to the necessity for a comprehensive medical service, but that was as far as it was prepared to go.

The Parliamentary Conservative Party had fired all its broad-sides without scoring a direct hit and even if it had the Labour Party's majority was such that it would have made no difference. Most of the consultants had made up their minds to join the service, so had the dental surgeons, the opticians and the pharmacists. The B.M.A. was aware of all these facts. Surely now the time had come for the general practitioners to start work in the N.H.S. on 5th July, 1948. But the B.M.A's hands were tied by the overwhelming majority opposed to such a decision as revealed by the plebiscites; now there must be yet another one. This time the B.M.A. set itself targets, one of which was that it would require 13,000 general practitioners out of a total of 20,000 to be opposed to cooperating with the service to make it unworkable. In the event the number fell well short of the target, only 9,588 general practitioners voted against accepting service under the Act.[19]

Within a few days of the result the B.M.A. recommended that the profession should "cooperate in the new service on the understanding that the Minister will continue negotiations on outstanding matters including terms and conditions of service for consultants and specialists, general practitioners, public health officers and others".[20]

And so it came about that the Medical profession agreed to start work on 5th July, 1948, in a service described by Aneurin Bevan as one "wherein medical treatment and care should be made available for rich and poor alike in accordance with medical need and by no other criteria".[21]

Epilogue

It has been alleged that the medical profession's attitude towards Aneurin Bevan during negotiations was hostile and that it remained so long after its introduction. Further, it has been alleged that the profession never gave him the credit he deserved for shaping and introducing the N.H.S. Perhaps there is some truth in these allegations although those who were close to him in the years of negotiation had a high opinion of his ability and almost all agreed that he had considerable personal charm. But some of his verbal outbursts upset people. One which was never entirely forgotten (or forgiven in some quarters) was the speech he made on the eve of the introduction of the N.H.S. in which he described the humiliation of the unemployed of the 1930's who were subjected to the Means Test.[22] "As far as I am concerned" he said, inter alia, "The Tory Party are lower than vermin". The speech offended a wide cross-section of the public and provided fuel for the Tory Press; so much so that it earned him a private but stern rebuke from the Prime Minister, Clement Atlee. Despite this he gradually won the

19. *"History of the B.M.A.," E. Gray Turner and F.M. Sutherland. Vol. II*
20. *Ibid.*
21. *"National Health Service, The First 30 years", Brian Abel-Smith.*
22. *More correctly "The Household Needs Test" in which a panel of lay investigators sometimes displayed a lack of sensitivity when inquiring into family savings or income from the un-employed man's wife or children, any one of which might result in the reduction of his dole.*

respect of the whole or almost the whole of the Medical profession and there is no doubt that in time his reputation was enhanced by comparison with some of his successors.

Although many eminent politicians trod the corridors of power of the Ministry of Health (later the Department of Health and Social Security), some inevitably left a better impression on the doctors than others; some left no impression at all. Among the former was Kenneth (later Sir Kenneth) Robinson, who was the son of a general practitioner.

Forty years on, viewed dispassionately, the main actors in the drama of the making of the N.H.S. were undoubtedly the B.M.A. and Aneurin Bevan. Each fought a good fight for their principles. The B.M.A. saved the doctors from a whole-time salaried state service which they feared would be the cornerstone of the N.H.S., and Bevan had the wisdom to agree to them being independant contractors to the government through the agency of Executive Councils. In addition he had the foresight and wisdom to unify the hospital system under central government and had the political courage to allow both general practitioners and consultants to have private patients. His contribution was immense; it would be mean for anyone to deny this. It was his greatest achievement, but it was to be his last. In 1951 when he was no longer Minister of Health[23] he resigned from the Cabinet over the introduction of charges for spectacles and dentures and the threat of prescription charges. He felt that his beloved Health Service was being unfairly singled out for economies which were to help to pay for increased expenditure on defence. Later that year the Conservative Party was back in power and for the remainder of his political life, which was to be the same as his life span,[24] Bevan was stranded in the affluent society.

REFERENCES

I would like to express my thanks to the following:

Lord Eden of Winton for permission to quote from *"Durham"* by his father Sir Timothy Eden, published by Robert Hale Ltd. 1952.

The Rt Hon Michael Foot P.C. M.P. for permission to quote from his book *"Aneurin Bevan 1945-1960"* published by Davis-Poynter Ltd 1973 and by Granada Publishing Ltd 1975.

William Heinemann Ltd for permission to quote from Lord Hill's autobiography *"Both Sides of the Hill,"* published 1964.

To the Controller of H.M.S.O. for permission to quote from *"National Health Service, The First Thirty Years."* by Prof. Brian Abel-Smith.

23. *Aneurin Bevan was Minister of Labour in the second post war Labour Government.*
24. *Aneurin Bevan died in 1960 aged 62.*

Mr. D.A. Parrott, Publishing Manager, the B.M.J., for permission to quote from *"History of the British Medical Association"* Vol. 11. 1932-1981, by E. Grey Turner and F M Sutherland, published by the B.M.A. 1982, and for permission to quote from the B.M.J. of 8/6/68.

BIBLIOGRAPHY

In addition to the above:

1. Gregg, Pauline *"A Social and Economic History of Britain, 1760-1972."* 7th Edition, Harrap 1972.
2. Seaman, L.C.B.*"Life in Britain between the Wars."* Batsford 1970.
3. Granshaw, Lindsay. *"Health for All."* (The Origins of the N.H.S. 1848-1948) Wellcome Institute for the History of Medicine. 1988.
4. Robinson, William. Sidelights on the life of a Wearside Surgeon 1859-1938, Northumberland Press Ltd., 1938.

A J A F

PART II

1948 Onwards

by

D T Prescott, M.B.B.S. FRCGP
Retired General Practitioner, Bishop Auckland.

1948 Onwards

The New Dawn

On the 5th July, 1948, the National Health Service was born and a new era commenced in the medical care of the population of the British Isles. Its aim was to take care of all the medical problems of the population without any financial liability to the patient. Overnight "The Panel" and the "Club System" disappeared. Every man, woman and child was given an opportunity of joining the Health Service and almost everyone took this opportunity, with the exception of a handful of private patients. The old Insurance Committee under "The Panel System" now became the Durham Executive Council covering the whole County. It was responsible for administrative arrangements for all the private contractors to the Health Service namely the general practitioners, the dentists, the opticians and the chemists. All patients wishing to register with a doctor had to fill in form EC1, this to be signed by the doctor of their choice and then safely lodged with the Executive Council at Durham for registration. The National Health Service registration number on this form was the same as the old war time identity number. Remuneration of the doctor was of course based on the old per capita system of the National Health Insurance Act of 1911. To decide the payment per capita there was a central pool of money which was divided by the number of registered patients in the country and the size of this pool was decided by the Government. The only way to increase ones income was to increase the number of patients on ones List. There was no reward for quality of service (a defect which still bedevils the National Health Service), and in a community such as the Wear Valley and Sedgefield Council Districts where the population was static, doctors were by common consent underpaid and overworked. Although immediately following the 5th July, 1948, there was not much change in the style of practice, after a few months the public suddenly realised there was a Service that had all the appearances of being free at the point of contact (despite the fact they were paying for it at that time with an Insurance Stamp). They realised that corsets, wigs, various appliances, bandages, cotton wool etc. were now all free. The flood gates opened, the patients poured in, the surgery sessions hitherto about one and a half hours duration expanded to about three hours, and the requests for home visits increased proportionately. General Practitioners, overwhelmed by the demand, sat back and wondered what had happened in the past to all the real and imaginary illnesses that the public now displayed. No longer was the general practitioner able to play golf in the afternoons, (a myth which still persists to this day). Most doctors at that time worked single handed, some had the luxury of an assistant or a partner, and if there was a partner it was usually a partnership of two. Anything more than that was indeed an exception, and a fortnight's holiday in the year was all that could be obtained and possibly afforded.

Whilst mentioning the supply of corsets, wigs etc. some of our readers may be interested to know a little facet of the new National Health Service. It was that an official Wig Repairer and Cleaner had to be appointed by the National Health Service. The only one with experience of this, over a wide area of the North of England, was a Mr Fred Thirkell, who before and just after the War kept a high class Ladies and Gents Hairdressers in the building in Bishop Auckland formerly occupied by Wades the House Furnishers. In those days wigs were made from natural hair and had to be very careully looked after. Apparently the only method of cleaning them, was for Mr Thirkell to take the wigs outside into the yard at the back of his premises and totally immerse them in petrol and hang them up to dry before he commenced to dress them, refurbish them and put the waves back in them.

In the period between the two World Wars, despite the formation of the Local Authority Mother and Child Services and the transfer of the old Poor Law Institutions to Local Authorities in late 1920s, many aspects of the British health care provision remained inadequate and the launch of the National Health Service was an effort to correct this. Many general practitioners felt that the division of some health services between general practices and local authorities was unsatisfactory. There was a considerable feeling that general practitioners worked in isolation and that practices were too small to offer flexibility and the range of services which the training and skills of doctors could provide. There were also unsurmountable problems in keeping up to date. Much of this was expressed by A J Cronin in his novel The Citadel which helped to bring the situation to public attention. The birth of the National Health Service in 1948 did little to improve this situation as we still had a tripartite service — a family practitioner service, a local authority health service and a hospital service. One major change, however, did take place. At the onset of the National Health Service in 1948 there was a separate Maternity Medical Service in which Doctors could agree to take part or not, and people had to register separately for this service with any Doctor of their choice, although most of them chose to have their own general practitioner. This was an individual contract for one confinement only, and the doctor was paid a special fee for this service. The result of this was that most practices set up their own ante natal clinics on a certain day of the week, and the patients rapidly accepted this Service and preferred it to pre 1948 conditions. From the onset of their pregnancy they were able to consult a doctor whom they knew and trusted, who was going to be responsible for the whole of their maternity care with the ability to refer for specialist consultation or hospital confinement where necessary.

Of the many problems of that time the distribution of doctors was extremely uneven throughout the country. In richer localities it was possible for family doctors to obtain a reasonable income, but in other localities this was far from the case, and it is interesting to note than an important Government Committee (Spens Committee) reported on General Practice remuneration in the late 1930s, and stated that "the percentage of low income (general practitioner) was too high, and unless conditions were substantially improved the social and economic status and recruitment of general practitioners would not be maintained! Under the 1946 National Health Service Act general practitioners retained their status of independent contractors to the Government (they are not employed by the Government) and together with a community based dental, pharmaceutical and optical service, all of whom are independent contractors, they form a separate division of the tripartite National Health Service structure. Each individual doctor, pharmacist, dentist and optician had a contract with the Durham Executive Council which administered all primary care services provided under the National Health Service Act. In addition to the responsibility of paying its contractors each Executive Council had a number of other duties, one of which was to appoint doctors to single handed practice vacancies.

Where there was a partnership of course the existing partners had the right to choose their own partner and do so to this day, but in addition the Executive Council had to supervise the supply of doctors dependent on classifications of practice areas. All areas of the country are classified according to the list sizes of the doctors. They were either designated areas, open areas, intermediate areas or restricted areas. Designated areas have the highest number of patients per doctor and restricted areas have the least number of patients per doctor. So you can well imagine there were very few restricted areas in the North of England and certainly none in the South West Durham area. There are now no designated areas in the country, but at one time Bishop Auckland, Spennymoor and Ferryhill were all designated areas. In point of fact Spennymoor and Ferryhill were among the last areas within the country to have their designation removed. If a doctor or doctors practising in intermediate areas wished to take a further partner then this would have to be referred to a committee, (a nine member independent body known as the Medical Practices Committee which was established under the 1946 Act,) with good reasons as to why this partnership should be allowed to have another doctor. It is interesting to note that amongst the nine members were two local practitioners, Dr P V Anderson of Shildon and Dr Fenwick Lishman of Crook. New partners could be taken into designated areas and open areas without any reference to the Medical Practices Committee, but entry to intermediate areas was certainly regulated by the Medical Practices Committee.

Years of Crisis

The first few years of the National Health Service had sapped the morale of general practitioners. Their income was nowhere near what they thought it ought to be, the workload was heavy and recruitment to general practice poor. However, 1952 was an interesting year for general practice. The first thing that happened was that the general practitioners went to arbitration about their remuneration, Mr Justice Dankwerts was approved as the Arbitrator both by the profession via the British Medical Association and the Government of the day. When arbitration was about to take place there was a General Election and a change of Government and the new Government also agreed to Mr Justice Dankwerts as the Arbitrator. The Profession therefore had a unique situation of both Government and Opposition agreeing to the same Arbitrator, and both sides of the House were left virtually speechless when something in the region of a 25% increase backdated to 1948 was awarded. The name of Mr Justice Dankwert, now long since could employ their own staff and the Government would repay substantial percentage of their wages up to a maximum of two whole time equivalents per Principal. This meant one could employ increased reception staff and also a Practice Nurse should one so wish.

The Charter also introduced a system of seniority payments for Doctors. These were awarded in three different stages depending on the number of years since a Doctor came onto the Medical Register after qualification, and also on the number of years in which he had been a Principal in General Practice. These factors varied as the Doctor became progressively older and of course the third stage seniority award was the highest award. The reasoning behind this was that as Doctors approached retiring age they might wish to take a lesser share of work in the Practice and also relinquish part of their share to the Juniors and to be compensated by their seniority award and retain the same level of income.

Improved Educational Facilities

In 1968 a report on medical education was published by a Committee under the Chairmanship of Professor Todd. Evidence had been taken from the General Medical Services Committee of the British Medical Association and the Royal College of General Practitioners leading to recommendations for vocational training in general practice, and the establishment of postgraduate councils for medical education. As a result of this, various vocational training schemes were set up in the country, and certain practices established as training practices. To become vocationally trained after completing compulsory pre-registration hospital jobs, the doctors then embarked on a three year course of vocational training, one year of which was spent in a training practice which could well mean two separate six months in two different practices. After the initial six months in practice there was then a series of four six month jobs in hospitals as a senior house officer. One of these had to be in medicine, one in paediatrics, one in obstetrics and gynaecology and the fourth one was variable and often something of the doctor's own choice, but as often as not it was psychiatry. Then they came back into a training practice for the final six months. At the end of that time most of them took the examination of the Royal College of General Practitioners for Membership of that College. In 1976 legislation was introduced to make vocational training mandatory for general practice as from 1982. So we have the situation today that no doctor can become a principal in general practice unless they have undertaken the three years vocational training scheme. One of the reasons for a vocational training scheme was that before the Second World War the newly qualified doctor was allowed to go immediately into practice. However, today general practitioners have to deal with the effects on people of the more complex society in which we all live. Complexity has created many personal, social and medico social problems which can give rise to symptoms, the cause of which is not easily or quickly diagnosed and the treatment of which may require recourse to a wide variety of medical and Social Services which have to be coordinated by the general practitioner. Medical technology has also advanced rapidly and this has two consequences for the general practitioner. In the first place he needs more time to keep abreast of developments and appreciate what they mean for patients. Secondly the increased need for the Consultant to concentrate on technology puts the onus more and more on the General Practitioner to carry the human aspect of medicine and explain matters to his Patients, who are more educated in medical matters than they used to be in the past. All this cannot be comprssed into the five years of Undergraduate Education where all the Specialities compete for time in the teaching process and therefore it is hoped to remedy these deficiencies during the Vocational Training Course and to produce a high calibre of doctor in general practice. As would be expected, the use of computers comprises part of the vocational training course and these have been introduced into many practices today. One of the particular uses is the recording, checking and issuing of repeat prescriptions.

All of this naturally led to gradual improvement in surgery premises, and additional staff being employed by doctors helped them to introduce such things as appointment systems. Employment of a practice nurse was also introduced in many practices, increasing the facilities available within the practice. The numbers of partnerships began to flourish and of course with the basic practice allowance applying to every principal it was possible to introduce new Partners into a Practice without severe detriment to the income of the other Partners.

Another development since the Family Doctors Charter was an increased use of deputising services. Although deputising services are not available in South West Durham, they may be in the future. The amalgamation of practices and increasing partners meant that the percentage of doctors on call for five or more nights in a week fell from 39% in 1964 to 9% in 1977, and in the Country as a whole about half the doctors use a deputising service.

At this stage one could say a few words about continued education which concerns the General Practitioners of South West Durham just as much as those in the rest of the Country. In the 1950's and 1960's a great deal of discussion took place between the British Medical Association and the Government and the Royal College of General Practitioners which highlighted the fact that education in general practice needed to be conducted at three levels; at the undergraduate stage, before entry into practice, and in the years of practice as a principal.

In South West Durham there had always been some form of postgraduate education, the original responsibility being that of the local division of the British Medical Association who at their meetings during the year used to invite speakers to come from the Newcastle Hospitals, particularly the Royal Victoria Infirmary — which was the University Teaching Hospital — to give lectures at their meetings. In addition after the advent of the appointment of consultants to the Bishop Auckland General Hospital following the advent of the National Health Service in 1948, a teaching

Some well known general practitioners of the past.

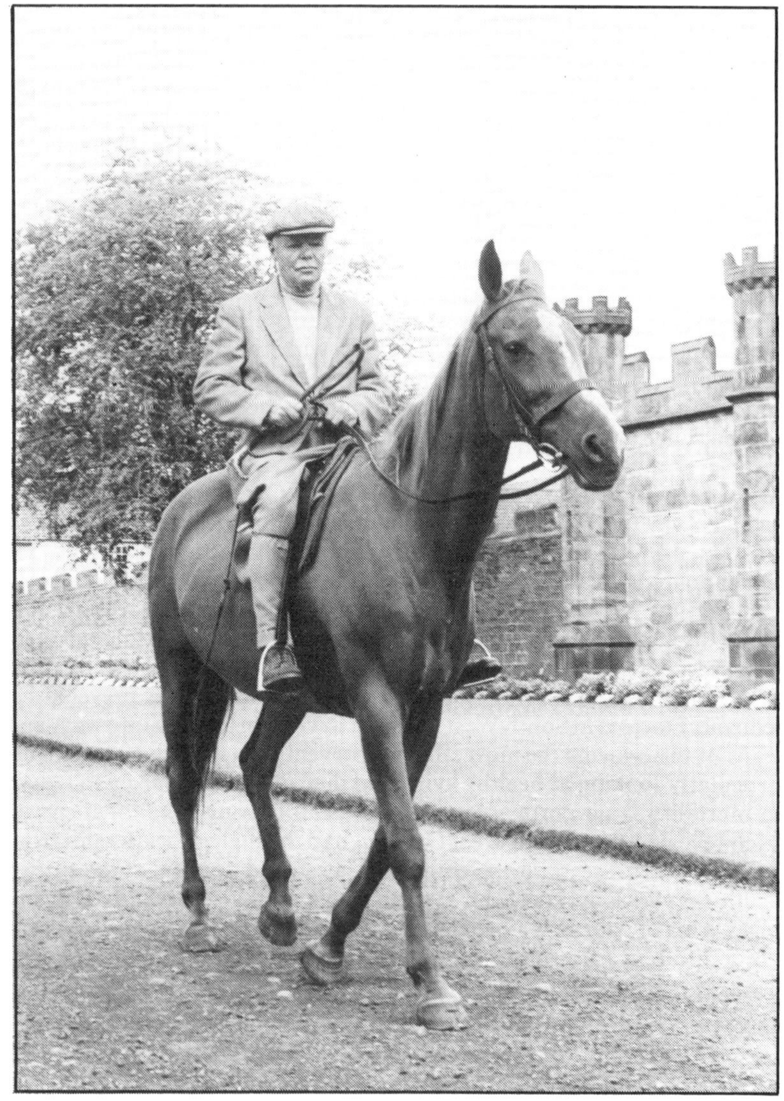

Dr V.H. Wardle of Bishop Auckland riding in the Bishop of Durham's Park.

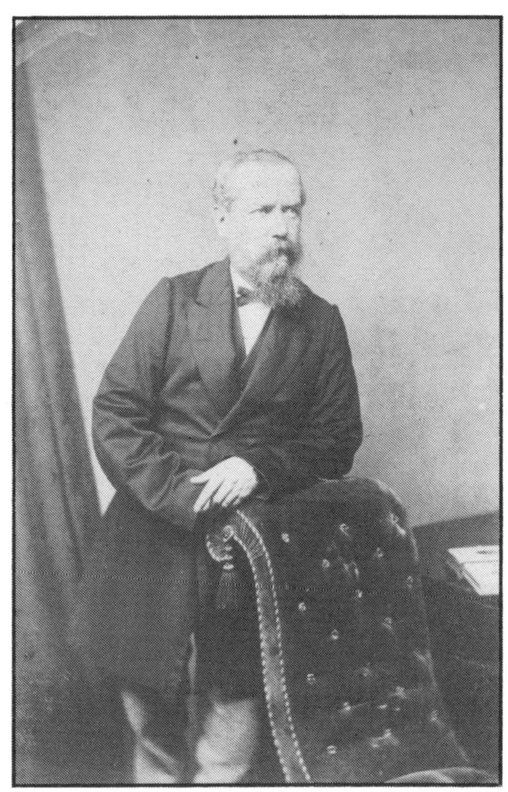

Dr Valentine Hutchinson of Bishop Auckland.

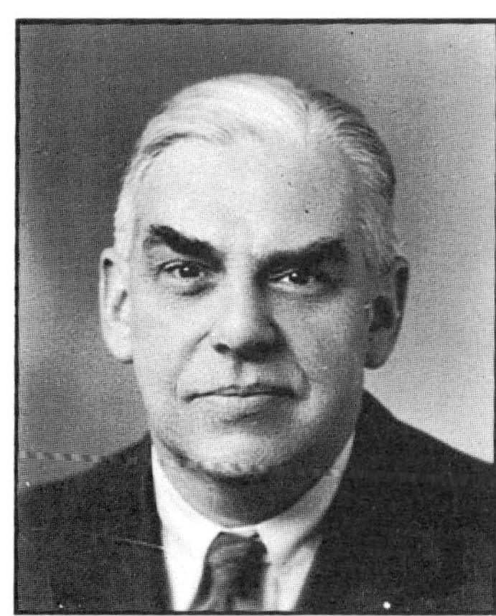

Dr P.V. Anderson of Shildon

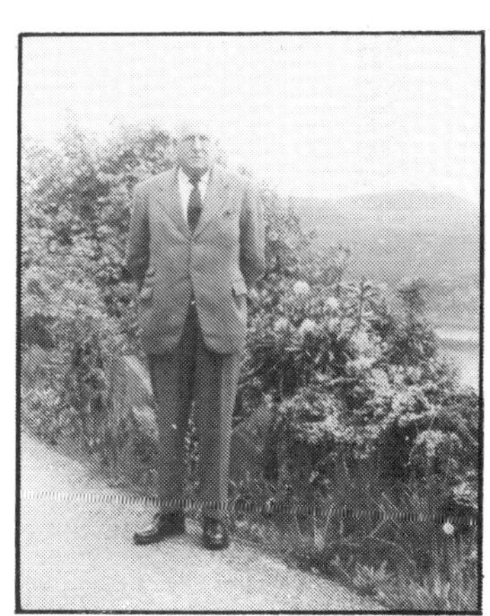

Dr A.C.H. McCullagh of Bishop Auckland.

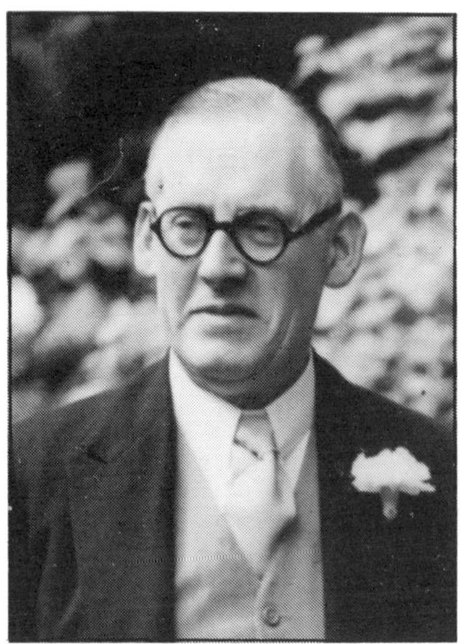
Dr Fenwick Lishman of Crook,

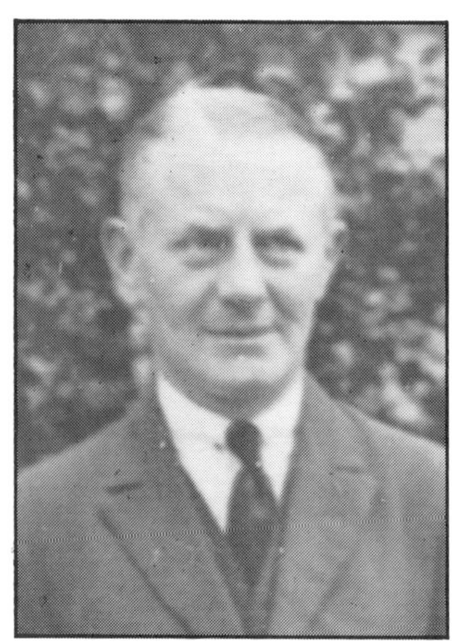
Dr T.E. Ferguson of Bishop Auckland.

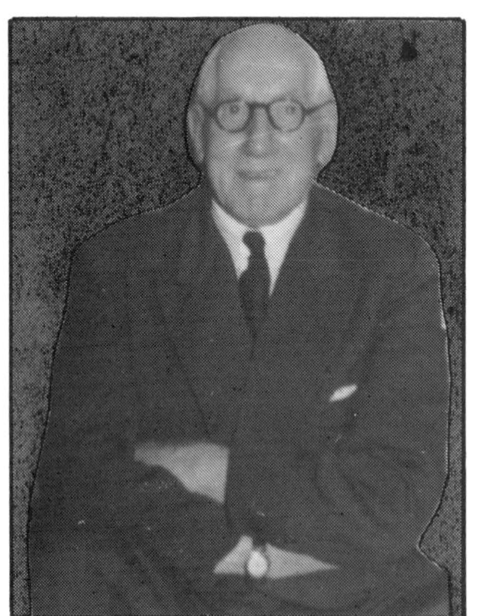
Dr William Anderson of Coundon

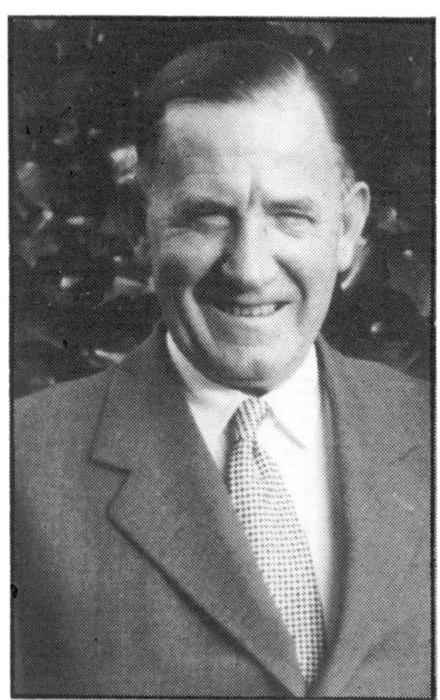
Dr S.E.H. Anderson of Cockfield.

PART III

The Origins of the General Practices in the S.W. Durham Health District

by

A.J.A. Ferguson and D.T. Prescott

Introduction

It would not have been possible to write a history of the general practices in this part of South West Durham without the co-operation of the families of former colleagues and of our present day colleagues who have been very helpful with information about their predecessors but very modest about themselves. Occasionally we have taken the liberty of adding items of interest such as war-time service and military decorations.

In tracing the origins of the general practices in the S.W. Durham Health District we have included those in Evenwood, Cockfield and Butterknowle although strictly speaking they are within the Darlington Health District. In the time span with which we are mainly concerned it is probably true to say that these practices were more closely linked with Bishop Auckland than with Darlington, but it is recognised that there is a flow of patients across all health districts.

The practices have been taken in alphabetical order starting with the town or village and the name of the first known doctor in each practice.

Bishop Auckland

Dr G.W. Ellis' Practice. Successors: Dr A.C. Farquharson, Dr G.R. Ellis, Dr T.E. Ferguson, Dr A.J.A. Ferguson, Dr D.T. Prescott, Dr C. Walne, Dr R. McManners, Dr I. Robertson, Dr G. Bolton, Dr L. McHugh, Dr N.L. Wilson.

This practice was established in 1879 by Dr G.W. Ellis with surgery accommodation at his house then known as Tenby House, now probably 28, 30 and 32 High Bondgate. Later he moved to the Elms in the Market Place which at one time had been the home of Dr V. Hutchinson. (q.v.) Dr Ellis was killed in an accident in Newgate Street in 1902 when driving his pony and trap and he was succeeded by Dr A.C. Farquharson.

When Dr Ellis' son G.R. (Reggie) Ellis qualified as a doctor in 1910 he joined the practice in partnership with Dr Farquharson who subsequently left to go into general practice in Spennymoor. Dr Reggie Ellis joined the R.A.M.C. in 1914 but he did not survive the war. After 1914 the practice was looked after by several locum tenens amongst whom were Dr D Miller and Dr S.J. Leonard until 1919 when Dr T.E. Ferguson bought the practice from Dr G.W. Ellis' widow. Before the war Dr Ferguson had been an assistant to Dr Mark Wardle and then in partnership with Dr William Anderson at Coundon where he lived in The Old Hall, Wharton Street which was approximately where numbers 30, 31 and 32 now stand. During the 1st World War he served in the R.A.M.C. as a Regimental Medical Officer in France.

In his early years in Bishop Auckland Dr Ferguson's surgery was at his house, 3 Victoria Street, but in 1923 the family and the surgery accommodation moved to Braeside, in the Market Place, appropriately enough next door to The Elms. The partnership with Dr William Anderson at Coundon continued for a while but as both practices gradually grew apart it was amicably dissolved in 1926. There-after Dr Ferguson had the help of a number of assistants the best remembered of whom are Dr Elizabeth Clark, Dr N.S. Hendry, Dr Sheila Murray, (who later went on to be Director of the Regional Blood Transfusion Service) and Dr J H O'Callaghan.

Dr T.E. Ferguson was one of a number of outstanding general practitioners in the area in the years between the wars. He had a flair for clinical medicine and was very considerate to his assistants and staff, and his ready wit often enlivened professional and social occasions. His retirement in 1948 was followed all too quickly by his death that same year.

He had been succeeded on his retirement by his son Dr A.J.A. Ferguson and Dr D.T. Prescott both of whom were his assistants after being in H.M. Forces in which Dr Prescott had served with distinction in the R.A.M.C. in Europe and Palestine. He was mentioned in despatches as well as being decorated by the Czechoslovakian Government for outstanding service to Czech national incarcerated in the concentration camp at Belsen; this decoration is equivalent to our D.S.O.

The surgery accommodation remained at Braeside until 1954 by which time it was clear that it was not big enough to cope with the expanding work load and it was moved to 37 Cockton Hill Road which was adapted to provide the necessary rooms and offices. Whilst there the partnership grew when Dr Colin Waine joined the practice in 1961, followed by Dr Robert McManners in 1975. In 1977 the practice headquarters were moved to accommodation in the newly built Health Centre in Escomb Road. Dr Ian Robertson joined the partnership in 1982 and Dr Gordon Bolton in 1983. When Dr Ferguson and Dr Prescott retired in 1986 after thirty eight years in partnership Dr Loretto McHugh who had been with the practice for a year became a partner; her unavoidable resignation in 1987 was due to her husband's unexpected move to a post in the South of England. She was succeeded by Dr Nigel Wilson that same year.

Bishop Auckland

Dr V. Hutchinson's Practice; Successors: Dr M.A. Wardle, Dr V.H. Wardle and Dr E.A. Fox.

The precise date of Dr Valentine Hutchinson's arrival in Bishop Auckland is uncertain, but it was before 1848, the year in which he was married.

Dr and Mrs Hutchinson lived first in 59 North Bondgate, later moving to The Elms in the Market Place. One of Dr Hutchinson's assistants was Dr Mark Wardle, who came to Bishop Auckland in 1870 and soon became engaged to Dr Hutchinson's daughter Jane. After a period of further study at Medical School in Newcastle and a period as an assistant in a practice there he returned to Bishop Auckland in 1880 married Miss Hutchinson and joined his father-in-law's practice as a partner, succeeding him on his retirement. At about this time the surgery accommodation moved to the old pink walled cottages, now demolished, on the north side of the Market Place. Dr and Mrs Mark Wardle lived first in No. 4 Belvedere, later moving to a house in Castle Square which subsequently was demolished to make way for Durham Road to emerge into the Market Place. From here he moved to nearby Silver Street, now known as King Street, and although he had a consulting rom there the main surgery accommodation remained in the cottages in the Market Place.

He was a versatile doctor capable of carrying out major surgical operations and he wrote several papers which were published in medical journals. By all accounts he was a forthright man who brooked no nonsense especially from the lay authorities with whom he had to deal in the course of his duties as Medical Officer to the Poor Law which included being in charge of the Infirmary at Oaklands, perhaps better known by its rather chilling name, The Workhouse.

Dr Mark Wardle was joined by his son Dr Valentine Hutchinson Wardle in 1913. Val Wardle, as he was affectionately known, was in general practice, apart from Army Service, until his retirement in 1966. He served in the R.A.M.C. in the 1914-18 war in which he won the Military Cross and again in the 1939-45 war in which he endured three and a half years as a prisoner-of-war of the Japanese during which time the family suffered a grevious loss when his son Tony was killed whilst serving in the Royal Air Force.

Dr Mark Wardle died in 1927 and Dr Val Wardle carried on the practice first from "Stanley House" and later from "Thornfield", both in Etherley Lane. During his absence in the 1939-45 war the practice was looked after by Dr A. Gaiter who continued as an assistant until 1948. In 1950 Dr Wardle was joined by his brother-in-law Dr G. Bickmore after whose departure in 1951 Dr E.A. Fox joined him in partnership. The following year the surgery accommodation moved to Dr Fox's house, "Craddock House", 25 Cockton Hill Road.

Dr Val Wardle held many appointments; he had succeeded his father as Medical Officer to the Poor Law which included being in charge of the Infirmary within Oaklands until the advent of the N.H.S. in July 1948. In addition he was at one time or another Police Surgeon, Treasury Medical Officer, Factory Act Medical Officer, and Medical Officer to the 6th Battalion, The Durham Light Infantry. He was an accomplished horseman and hunted with the South Durhams and was Honorary Surgeon to both the South Durham and Zetland Point to Point. His partnership with Dr Fox lasted until his retirement in 1966 when Dr Fox entered into a new partnership with Dr A.H. Dawes and Dr I.G. Lloyd and with Dr S.K. Young.

When Dr Val Wardle died in 1968 the affection in which he was held by the people of Bishop Auckland was perfectly summed-up in this extract from his obituary written by Dr Fox and published in the British Medical Journal:

"Val Wardle was greatly respected by all who knew him. One of the best known personalities in Bishop Auckland, he was a man of principle and integrity with a delightful sense of humour and quick wit. Brisk in manner and step and alert in mind until the day of his death, he had a kindness for his patients which they greatly appreciated and a remarkable knowledge of them and their family histories."

Bishop Auckland

The Practice of Drs T.A. and A.C.H. McCullagh.

Dr T.A. McCullagh came to Bishop Auckland as assistant to Dr G.W. Ellis and later established his own practice in Clarendon House, Newgate Street, a house now demolished but which was near the Wesleyan Church. His son Dr Cecil McCullagh joined the practice before the First World War in which he served with distinction in the R.A.M.C. being awarded the D.S.O. Dr Cecil McCullagh's wife was the daughter of Dr Kane of Byers Green, who after his retirement lived in The Towers, Etherley Lane. In the early 1920's Dr T.A. McCullagh moved to 11, The Market Place, but the practice headquarters continued to be at Clarendon House.

Dr T.A. McCullagh is amongst a group of doctors referred to in Sir Timothy Eden's book "Durham":[1]

"And here come the doctors with no thoughts of "nationalisation" in their robust and independent hearts. Dr Hind of Norton on his chestnut mare; Dr McCullagh of Bishop Auckland, who loved Balzac and his clinking brown hunter; Dr Fenwick of Chilton Hall, with a cheery word and a glass of orange brandy for the huntsmen after a hard day."

Dr Cecil McCullagh was a kindly man, and a popular figure in the town. There were several lady assistants in the practice amongst whom were Dr McFadyean, Dr Foster, Dr M. Hegarty and Dr Moore.

When Dr Cecil McCullagh retired in 1946 the practice was amalgamated with Dr V H Wardle's practice.

1. *"Durham", Sir Timothy Eden, Vol II p.443.*

Bishop Auckland, Close House.

Dr J. Mason's Practice. Successors: Dr J.B.D. Oliver, Dr A.H. Dawes, Dr I.G. Lloyd.

Dr J. Mason was in practice in Close House, Eldon and Eldon Lane from about 1900 until the 1930s. He lived in Close House and in his early years he did his visiting rounds in a trap drawn by a highly intelligent horse. History has it that the horse required no direction in taking the doctor on his rounds from Close House to Eldon, on to Eldon Lane and then back to Close House again with occasional excursions into Auckland Park. Dr Mason was a figure of great importance in the mining community and his visits to the homes of the sick were viewed with trepidation allied to a feeling of relief that he was in charge of the case.

He was joined in the early 1930's by Dr J.B.D. Oliver, one of four doctor brothers who practised in County Durham. Dr Basil Oliver was a kindly man with a forceful personality, who became well known and respected in the area. After Dr Mason retired in the late 1930's Dr Oliver ran the practice on his own until 1946 when Dr Short joined him as his assistant. Dr Short was succeeded by Dr Harry Dawes in 1949 who soon became a partner and in 1957 the surgery accommodation increased from the practice headquarters in Close House, with a branch surgery in Coundon, to include purpose built accommodation in Dr Dawes newly built house in Woodhouse Lane. At about this time Dr Charles Diamond now a well known, Ear, Nose and Throat Surgeon in Newcastle was an assistant in the practice.

The closure of pits in Leasingthorne, Auckland Park and Eldon led to the migration of a large number of miners and their families to Nottingham and the Midlands, and at the same time Durham County Council decided that development of the pit villages around Bishop Auckland should not continue and that they should be allowed to run down. The focus of new council house building was now in the town of Bishop Auckland itself with the majority of it concentrated in the Woodhouse Close Estate and it was to this estate that many of Dr Oliver's and Dr Dawes' patients moved. In 1961 the partners were joined by a nephew of Dr Oliver, Dr Ian Lloyd, whose father, grandfather and great-grandfather were doctors. Dr Ian Lloyd's son Christopher is also a doctor making the fifth generation in the family, a remarkable record. Following the death of Dr Oliver in 1962 and the amalgamation of the practice with those of Dr Sandy Fox and Dr Sam Young in 1967 the combined practices moved to new accommodation at 83 Cockton Hill Road, Bishop Auckland.

Prior to this Dr Dawes and Dr Lloyd had begun negotiations concerning the planning of the Health Centre in Coundon to replace their existing surgery accommodation there. Dr Steele, who was also in practice in Coundon at that time, was approached about accommodation in the proposed Health Centre and as a result the plans included consulting suites for both practices. It was also to include Community Health Service clinics and after a lengthy gestation period it was ready for use by November 1975. With regard to their Bishop Auckland surgery accommodation the partners moved in 1978 from 83 Cockton Hill Road to the newly built Health Centre in Escomb Road.

Dr Prudence Beckingham was a partner during the 1970's and when she left she was succeeded by Dr Dawes' son-in-law Dr Jan Freeman who wished to obtain experience in general practice. He left to resume his hospital career a year later and is now a consultant physician and gastro-enterologist in Derby City Hospital. He was succeeded by Dr Marion McEvoy who was with the practice until 1978 when she left to take up an appointment in Community Medicine. She was succeeded by Dr B.R. Pike who had spent some years in general practice in Australia and New Zealand. Dr G.S. McGregor joined the practice in 1981 when Dr Fox retired after 30 years in general practice in Bishop Auckland. Dr S. Findlay joined the practice in 1984 and in 1988 Dr P. Bowron and Dr Mary Carney joined the partnership. Later that year Dr Dawes retired after 39 years in the practice and Dr Young after 27 years as a partner of the late Dr Leslie and in the present partnership.

Bishop Auckland, Eldon

Dr G. Thorpe's Practice. Successors: Dr T. Fraser, Dr J. Leslie, Dr S.K. Young.

This practice was established in about 1900 with surgery accommodation in Dr Thorpe's house on Eldon Bank. He was succeeded by his son-in-law Dr Fraser who on his retirement in 1946 was succeeded by Dr John Leslie. By this time the doctor's home and the surgery accommodation had moved to Coronation Villa, Coronation.

John Leslie qualified in Glasgow and served in the R.A.M.C. during the 2nd World War. He was a hard working and deservedly popular general practitioner. He was joined in partnership by Dr S.K. Young in 1961, before which he had a number of assistants, the best remembered of whom are Dr M. Gorzenski, Dr Betty K. Dean, and Dr Ann Ropner.

Sadly, John Leslie died prematurely in 1965. Such was the affection in which he was held by his patients that they refurbished a ward in the Lady Eden Hospital to his memory. The practice was carried on by Dr S K Young with the help of his wife Dr Jean Young until the amalgamation with the practices of Drs Dawes and Lloyd and Dr Fox in 1966.

Bishop Auckland, Witton Park

Dr McKechnie's Practice. Successors: Dr Williamson, Dr Cuncliffe, Dr T.F. Heas, Dr D.B. Cama, Dr L. Cama, Dr J. Clark, Dr H. Shuttleworth, Dr A. Lewis, Dr D. Harris, Dr C.M. Scott, Dr A. McLeod, Mr D.F. Gallagher and Dr M.A. Ward.

The first recorded Doctor in that area was Dr McKechnie, somewhere around 1850, and it is interesting to note that one of his children was baptised in the Saxon Church at Escomb in 1863, and there is a memorial window to Dr McKechnie in St. Paul's Church, Witton Park. Dr McKechnie was followed by Dr Williamson, who died in 1898, to be followed by Dr Cunliffe who died in November, 1915, and who was followed by Dr T.F. Heas. Sometime in the early 1920's Dr D.B. Cama succeeded Dr Heas, Dr Cama having been an assistant in Bishop Auckland with Mr Mark Wardle. In the early 1930's he bought Dr Heslop's practice whose surgery was in Clyde House in Gibbon Street, Bishop Auckland. Dr Cama came to live in Bishop Auckland in the house which is now the Cockton Hill Branch of Barclays Bank and Dr Heslop went to Witton Park as his assistant. Dr Cama was joined in practice by his son Dr Leonard Cama in 1945 following service in the Royal Navy during the War. Meanwhile there had been a succession of assistants at Witton Park living at Carwood House, which still has its speaking tube from the bedroom to the front door, and in 1947 Dr H.J. Shuttleworth arrived as the last assistant in the practice at Witton Park and at a later date became a partner. Following Dr Heslop there were a series of assistants at Witton Park, one of whom was Dr Momand, who apparently was of Dutch origin, and the other was Dr Harold Morck, who was Dr D.B. Cama's brother-in-law, he stayed in Witton Park a short while and took a practice of his own at Sowerby Bridge in Yorkshire. The last assistant prior to Dr Shuttleworth was Dr Walker.

Dr D.B. Cama retired in 1949 by which time the practice headquarters were at 54 Cockton Hill Road. Dr John Clark joined the practice in 1950, and Dr Alan Lewis in 1959.

Dr Leonard Cama took early retirement from practice in 1978 and went to live in the Lake District, where he continued his medical career as an anaesthetist and in 1969 Dr David Harris joined the practice, and in 1976 Dr Angus MacLeod joined the partnership.

Dr John Clark retired from the practice in 1984 and Dr Gallagher became a partner in 1985, and within recent months Dr M.A. Ward has joined the practice.

In 1966 an amalgamation took place with the West Auckland practice of Dr C.M. Scott, who had been practising on his own following the departure of Dr Grainger to Ferryhill, and he joined the partnership for a comparitively short while before joining the Department of Health and Social Security as a Regional Medical Officer.

And so the practice of Drs A. Lewis, D. Harris, A.H. MacLeod, D.F. Gallagher, and M.A. Ward, is a mixed urban and rural practice, originating in Witton Park in the mid-nineteenth century, with a main surgery still at 54 Cockton Hill Road, Bishop Auckland, and a second surgery, which was purpose-built comparatively recently, following the temporary amalgamation with Dr C.M. Scott's West Auckland practice, at 16 Manor Road, St Helens, West Auckland. The Witton Park surgery, of course, had closed some time around 1967.

Butterknowle and Copley

Dr Beattie' Practice. Successors: Dr Redmond, Dr Alexander, Dr A. Pearson, Dr D. Wright, Dr M. Clay, Dr G. Mees and Dr J. Pickworth.

Dr Michael Clay, now retired and living at Blencarne, near Penrith writes as follows:-

"In October 1961 I became assistant, and in 1962 a partner, to Dr Anthony Pearson of Butterknowle, and became what was known as "Copley Doctor". As such, I was one of a line living in the same house. The first was Dr Beattie, an Ulsterman. He combined general practice with farming and part of a field near the banks of the Gaunless was known as "Doctors Bottoms" (botham is old English for walking)."

For very many years after the Second World War, Dr Beattie still enjoyed a considerable reputation amongst his old patients. It was alleged he was able to diagnose Diphtheria by the smell as he entered the sick room. When he retired early in the Second World War he was succeeded by a Dr Redmond an Irish woman. From descriptions by her patients Dr Clay envisaged her as forthright, tweedy and fond of a "social glass". In 1947 she was succeeded by Dr Alexander who was a devout Christian and a total abstainer, and he was an accomplished preacher in the true Billy Graham tradition.

In 1954 he took Dr Anthony Pearson into partnership. Dr Pearson was a Rhodes scholar, and had been a medical missionary in Africa. It is reported that Dr Pearson, when once discussing medical cases with a consultant physician, who shall remain nameless, said very seriously that he once lost a patient, and then after a pause added, "To a lion!" Dr Alexander moved to Grassmere in 1959 and Dr David Wright was "Copley Doctor" until Dr Clay joined Dr Pearson in 1961. Dr Pearson, of course, practising from the Butterknowle end of the practice. Dr Pearson resigned in 1967 to join the School Health Service, when Dr Clay took over the practice and remained there for 17 years. These 17 years being marked by some interesting changes. Domiciliary obstetrics declined almost to extinction.

Dr Clay writes as follows:

"1961 home confinements were still numerous, by 1978 only the rare "rough" woman, or the rare "alternative" woman wished to be confined at home. The key to domiciliary obstetrics was the District Midwife, in our case Sister Mary Slack. These skillful women with their patience, care and practiced intuition, are probably irreplaceable.

These years 1961 to 1978 were also the time of the rise of drug induced diseases such as the thalidomide disaster.

In immunology, Smallpox vaccination sustained an overdue but well earned redundancy. Diphtheria and Poliomyelitis, the heart land of childhood immunisation programme, became virtually extinct, but not worldwide.

"The Pill" boosted a change in sexual morals. There were fewer unwanted pregnancies but more genito-urinary pathology.

Memorable idiosyncrasies of the practice were the high level of home visits and car boot dispensing and the severity and pessimism of snow fall."

There has been no "Copley Doctor" since Dr Pearson resigned in 1967 and Dr Clay continued the medical care of that area from the surgery at Butterknowle, and there is now no surgery at Copley. On 1st January 1979, Dr Graham Mees took over the practice from Dr Clay having been appointed by Durham F.P.C. some months earlier, and having completed a short service commission in H.M. Forces. More recently the Medical Practices Committee allowed Dr Mees to take in a partner, namely Dr Julia Pickworth.

Cockfield

Dr D.A. Anderson's Practice. Successors: Dr S.E.H. Anderson, Dr W. Neville, Dr I. Waller and Dr G.C. Slade.

The earliest known doctor in Cockfield is Dr D.A. Anderson who was born in Maghera, County Londonderry. He qualified in 1894 and before settling in Cockfield in 1896 was an assistant to Dr Neligan at Middleton-in-Teesdale. At first he lived in Church Square moving to Cockfield House in 1897. His elder son, Samuel Eric Hill Anderson (affectionately known to everyone as Sam) embarked on a medical career as a student in 1914 but volunteered for the army the following year and was commissioned in The Northumberland Fusiliers. He was wounded at the battle of the Somme in 1916 and following his discharge from the army on medical grounds in 1917 resumed his medical studies and qualified in 1921 when he joined his father's practice.

Dr D.A. Anderson died in 1923 and two or three years later Dr Sam Anderson moved to Woodview from where he practiced until he retired in 1960. Sam Anderson was a very popular and able general practitioner and looked after a widely scattered rural population as far afield from Cockfield as Woodlands and Staindrop where he had a branch surgery. His daughter Patricia remembers the great storm of 1947 when Cockfield was cut off from the surrounding towns and villages by deep snow drifts. She accompanied her father on foot from Cockfield to Staindrop being guided by the tops of the hedges and walls, sometimes walking above them. When Dr Anderson had seen the patients in the surgery and had done his rounds in the village they had some suitable refreshment in The Black Swan and walked back to Cockfield.

The Anderson family played a full part in the life of the local community. Dr D.A. Anderson was a County Councillor for several years and Dr Sam Anderson played football for Cockfield, later becoming Chairman of the Football Club and subsequently the President. In addition he captained

Raby Castle Cricket Club for whom he was a very successful all-rounder. The family traidition in local government was continued by Dr Sam Anderson's wife Barbara who was the first lady Chairman of Barnard Castle Rural District Council besides being on the Cockfield Parish Council for many years.

During the second World War the family suffered a sad loss when Trevor, who was destined to take up a career in medicine after the war and to join his father in practice, was killed after the D-Day landings in Normandy in the assault on Caen.

In 1949 Dr William Neville joined Dr Anderson as a partner staying for about one year before going into practice with Dr Hickey at Gainford. In June 1955 Dr Idris Waller came as assistant and was made a partner in February 1956. Dr Sam Anderson retired in 1960 to nearby Winston where sadly he died the following year.

In 1972 Dr Geoffrey Slade* joined Dr Waller as a partner. The practice headquarters are still at "Woodview" with a branch surgery at The Old Vicarage, Staindrop and another at Swan Street, Evenwood.

* *Dr Geoffrey Slade died suddenly shortly before this book was published.*

Coundon

Dr William Anderson's Practice. Partners and Successors: Dr T.E. Ferguson, Dr R. Thorpe M.C., Dr W. Steele and Dr I.H. Taylor.

This practice was originally part of Dr Mark Wardle's practice in which both Dr W. Anderson and Dr T.E. Ferguson were assistants. Dr Anderson bought the practice in 1912 and although it is by no means certain, it seems likely that he also took over Dr Campbell's practice at about the same time, the latter having been in practice in Coundon for several years prior to this. The surgery accommodation was adjacent to his house, "Roseberry". He was in partnership at Coundon with Dr T.E. Ferguson until the latter took over Dr Ellis' practice in Bishop Auckland. Dr Roland Thorpe M.C. joined Dr Anderson in 1920 living in Collingwood Street until 1927 when he left to go into practice in Edinburgh. There-after there were several lady assistants in the practice amongst whom were Dr Jamieson, Dr Benson and Dr Christine Anderson who although of the same name was not a relative. Dr Steele joined Dr Anderson in 1947 and became a partner shortly afterwards and carried on the practice after Dr Anderson retired in 1957.

Dr William Anderson was a kindly Scotsman and a good clinician who served a mixed mining and rural community faithfully for forty five years. He was surgeon to Leasingthorne Colliery and gave valuable service there whenever called upon.

He was interested in the St. John's Ambulance Brigade and gave lectures in the winter months and examined the candidates for proficiency in first aid. He was keen on all sports particularly football and enjoyed a flutter on the horses especially any from Mr Arthur Stephenson's stables at Leasingthorne. In 1960 he retired to Scarborough where he died in 1963.

Dr I.H. Taylor joined Dr Steele in 1960 and they were in partnership until 1974 when Dr Taylor left to join the Ferryhill group practice.

Dr Willlam Steele was a quiet, undemonstrative Scotsman with a reputation for being especially attentive to the elderly patients in his practice. When he retired in 1975 the practice was amalgamated with that of Drs Ferguson, Prescott, Waine and McManners. Three months later the practice premises moved to the newly completed Health Centre in Victoria Road and over sixty years of general practice based on "Roseberry" came to an end, and for one member of the partnership, a family wheel had come full circle.

Coundon

Dr J.L.C. Lagois and Dr U.J. Cherry's Practice

Dr J.L.C. Lagois, who came from Trinidad, was a general practitioner in Coundon from 1919 to 1925 when he died at the early age of 36. Shortly after his arrival in Coundon he was joined by his friend Dr U.J. Cherry who took over the practice after his death.

Dr Urban Jules Cherry, who lived at 58 Wharton Street, was a well known and impressive figure in Coundon and Bishop Auckland. Born in Trinidad he qualifed at Edinburgh University and first practised in London. He was a popular and respected practitioner who expected his patients to carry out his instructions to the letter. He was especially considerate towards those who needed his attention but could ill afford to pay for it. He did not have a car and did his visiting rounds or foot or by public transport.

Both Dr Lagois and Dr Cherry played cricket for Bishop Auckland the latter being an all rounder of quite outstanding ability and a popular figure on all the grounds in the North Yorkshire and South Durham League. On his death in 1946 the practice ceased to exist, the care of his patients being taken over by other doctors in the district.

Crook

Dr Moor tells us that the first record of a medical practitioner in Crook which he had seen was in "Who's Who" for Durham County, mid 19th century, was an unqualified doctor living in Arthur Street, which was probably the fashionable area in those days (it still contains a few large houses), but that he couldn't recall his name.

Meanwhile the originator of the present practice of Drs Ferguson, Chesters, Clarke, Proud and Waldron, was a Dr Kelly, who came about 1870 and built "Palmfield House" in a field belonging to the Roman Catholic Church and hence the name.

As far as our records go a Dr Reid was the first occupier of the "Red House" the practice now being run by Dr A.K. Banerjee.

Dr H.G. Caldwell's Practice. Successors: Dr R. Parkin and Dr S. Parkin.

There was also a third practice about which little is known prior to the first World War, but this was owned at that time by a Dr G.Y. Caldwell. He was Chairman of the Bishop Auckland Division of the British Medical Association in 1921 and 1922. His practice was purchased by Drs Ralph and Sybil Parkin just after the Second World War and prior to the commencement of the Health Service in 1948. In 1951 they were succeeded by Dr George Pearson.

Dr Kelly' Practice. Successors: Dr A. Mackay, Dr F. Lishman O.B.E., Dr G. Miller, Dr J.C. Moor, Dr G. Pearson, Dr G. Ferguson, Dr E.W. Chesters, Dr J.A. Clarke, Dr J.J. Proud and Dr J.H. Waldron.

To return to the practice of Dr Kelly, some time about 1880 to 1890, he was succeeded by a Dr Alexander MacKay, also living at "Palmfield". He had two sons and one daughter, and built up a very considerable practice employing several assistants, who travelled each day to the outlying villages on horse back, returning to "Palmfield" at night. Most of them must have lived there because it was reported by Dr Fenwick Lishman, senior partner to Dr Moor, that Mrs MacKay used to padlock the assistants beer barrel at a stated time each night. One assistant became junior partner probably about 1914-1918, a Dr Carlson, who is still remembered by some of the very old patients of Crook. Dr MacKay had two sons, William and George, and William qualified in medicine and succeeded his father in the early 1920's. He apparantly had a "short fuse", and a wonderful flow of invective. He served in the South African War and and the 1914-18 War with distinction, and was seriously wounded. He was greatly respected and well liked by people in Crook, but he was never very interested in general practice, and seemed more concerned with hunting and a little farming, and in due course was succeeded by Drs Gavin Miller and Fenwick Lishman, on payment of a small annuity.

Dr Moore succeeded Dr Miller in 1932, and was told that he would have to be responsible for part of the annuity, that Dr MacKay was already 60 and in poor health, so obviously he need not worry much about the annuity. Dr Moor looked after him for some years after the 1939-45 War and he eventually died at about the age of 80.

There apparently had been two other doctors in the area, in the villages of Hunwick and Howden-le-Wear, and their houses are still distinguished by speaking tubes from the front door to the bedrooms.

It will now be interesting to everyone to have a verbatim report by Dr Moor following his arrival in Crook in 1932, on the conditions prevailing in practice from that time until his retirement.

"In August 1932, I arrived in Crook accompanied by a small dog, a Morris Minor (value £25) and roughly the same amount in the bank! Petrol was approximately one shilling per gallon, so I was able to survive as assistant for six weeks, then as junior partner in succession to Dr G Millar.

Our Surgery in "Palmfield" consisted of a downstairs consulting room, a combined waiting room and dispensary; a scullery with a spare cold tap and a small upstairs consulting room. This had originally been the stable block. It was not commodious and the waiting room queue frequently extended down Church Hill.

We subsequently removed to much better accommodation in North House, the old Rectory."

Dr Moor served in the Navy during the Second World War and during that time Dr Lishman was assisted by a Dr N.L. Cannon, and a Dr Cecelia Cleary (later Mrs Corrigan), and two Irish Doctors whose names cannot be remembered. During his Naval service Dr Moor was awarded the Greek War Cross by the Greek Government for service to the Allied cause, Dr Moor was serving in H.M.S. Calcutta, when she was lost during the evacuation of Crete.

Dr George Pearson arrived in Crook on Whit Saturday, 1948 having spent three years in the Army and in partnership in Silksworth for one year. He records that the very next morning at 8.30, he was called to deliver a retained placenta for in those days domiciliary midwifery was the rule, with only anticipated difficulties and emergencies going to hospital. He records there was some hair raising moments but remarkably few catastrophies. For the first three years he was employed as an assistant to Drs Lishman and Moor at North House, Crook, and then in 1951 with the encouragement of his employers, he succeeded to the practice of Drs Ralph and Sybil Parkin at "Meadow House". This continued as an independent practice with about 2,250 patients supplemented with some of the following that Dr Pearson had acquired as an assistant at North House. In 1954 Dr Grant Ferguson who had not long completed his service in the Royal Air Force, and had just finished working as an assistant with a view to a partnership in a practice in West Auckland, which did not materialise, joined the Crook practice. Drs Lishman, Moor and Ferguson practiced from North House with Dr Pearson, the other partner practicing from Meadow House, and the patients considered themselves either Meadow House or North House patients and were very loath to go to the opposite surgery. This situation continued until Dr Lishman's retirement in 1965, when Dr Pearson left Meadow House and came to join the rest of the practice in North House in a truly amalgamated practice.

Drs Lishman and Moor had another assistant at the time of Dr Ferguson's arrival, a Dr Joseph, who was an expatriate Pole who had qualified at the Polish School of Medicine, which had transferred to Edinburgh during the War. He was much older than Dr Grant Ferguson, and was unsettled and was looking for a practice of his own. About this time he managed to get a vacancy near Sunderland.

In the years before Dr Lishman retired he was heavily involved in medical politics and was not only Chairman of Durham County Local Medical Committee, but he was also a Member of the General Medical Services Committee in London, whence he travelled almost every week. He was very much at the centre of things in London and very proud of his Membership of the Reform Club and friendship with the Home Secretary, Henry Brooke. All this was a far cry from doing night visits in the back streets of Crook. He had, of course, done his share of this, especially during the War, and even at this time used to go around Homelands Hospital at 7 a.m. before catching the morning train to London, and then do 10 to 15 visits in Witton-le-Wear on his way home from the evening Pullman. Just before he retired he was awarded an O.B.E. for his services to General Practice which gave him enormous pleasure. During his absence in London, Dr Fenwick Lishman gave Dr Grant Ferguson an opportunity to deputise for him in his capacity as Clinical Assistant in the day to day care at Homelands Hospital, Crook, and by now of course, Dr Grant Ferguson was a partner in the practice.

Homelands Hospital by this time was no longer a Fever Hospital, but had become a Geriatric Unit, now the acute fevers were becoming less serious and prevelent in the area. There was still one ward which was used for the overspill of tuberculosis from Holywood Hall, and although tuberculosis was no longer the serious problem it had been before and during the War, since the advent of Streptomycin, Dr Ferguson recalls that he was still in time to see a number of deaths in young people from massive haemoptysis.

At this point there is a verbatim quote from interesting facts that Dr Grant Ferguson gave us about the present Crook practice:

"Certainly the Asian 'flu epidemic of 1957 is one outstanding memory of my first few years in Crook. It started in September and went on for about 6 - 8 weeks before spluttering to a standstill in mid-November. The visiting level was extremely high at this time, and I did between 50 and 60 new calls daily for several weeks. I notice that Dr Moor does not think that this epidemic was as serious as the epidemic of 1933 - 1934, and he may well be right, but it was my impression that the population was fitter by 1957 and better equipped to deal with the disease; nevertheless, a number of people did die very rapidly from influenzal pneumonia, and it was also my impression that the geriatric problem was never as serious again after the epidemic had subsided.

Dr Lishman retired in 1965 and Dr Pearson came to join us in North House, and so for the first time the whole practice was under one roof.

Mr & Mrs Edward Goodfellow (and her old mother) lived on the top floor of the surgery, and took and passed on all the calls as they came in. Edward had been with Dr Lishman for many years, and was his chauffeur and right hand man, as well as helping with reception and dispensing. Monnie, his wife, was receptionist and dispenser, and the two of them did an enormous amount of work for the practice as partners. It is interesting to note that Dr Chesters now lives in, and has renovated "Palmfield", where the practice began.

The five of us continued like this for a number of years until Dr Moor decided to "wind down" and this enabled us to bring Dr J.A. Clarke into the practice following a spell as Medical Officer in the Royal Army Medical Corps.

The next major development in the history of the practice was the building of a new surgery. It had been our intention to work from a Local Authority Health Centre, but when we were told that no more funds would be made available for the building of a Health Centre, we grasped the bull by the horns and financed the building of a new surgery on a site in Hope Street.

This was done with some trepidation, because a large sum of money was involved, but in retrospect, of course, this has proved to be a very sound investment, and the older partners wonder why we did not do this years before. This has led to a great centralisation of the practice, because when I first came here, not only did we have two separate main surgeries in Crook, but there were either Call Houses or surgeries in all the surrounding villages, e.g. in Hunwick, Witton-le-Wear, Stanley, Roddymoor and Fir Tree, where calls could be left, patients seen and medicines dispensed. All these have now closed and the resistance of the patients to these moves has long since departed in the light of increased personal transport in the area. There is no doubt that this has led to a much more efficient use of resources. The whole style of the practice has gradually altered, and the visiting, although still I think a good deal higher than the national average, has fallen tremendously; on the other hand, with the advent of appointments in the surgery, the number of patients seen does not vary from month to month as it used to do, but remains at a fairly high level throughout the whole year, whereas it used to be much more seasonal.

Patients have altered as well in that in my early years, they consisted almost entirely of working men who were in the local pits or nearby heavy industry, and now there are no pits and there has been a fairly large influx of commuters into the new estates in the area.

The other striking change in my time in the practice has been the huge improvement in the standard of housing. In 1957 much of the housing was still very bad, particularly in Stanley, where a large proportion of the houses were still served by outside toilets, and many of the houses themselves were in a rundown condition. Since then there has been a huge programme of Council rehousing established and rehousing of the elderly in bungalow accommodation, and I suspect that the level of that is very high compared to the national average.

Dr Moor finally retired in 1980 and Dr G.D. Holbrook joined us as a partner, and then Dr Pearson followed him into retirement in April 1987, he in his turn being replaced by Dr J.J. Proud.We have just taken into partnership Dr J.H. Waldron, and I look forward to "winding down" in the next few years before I eventually retire, and so the practice goes on and continues to evolve.

It is interesting that Dr Moor, who still comes in to see us every week, provides a direct link with the earliest days of the practice, and I think that this gives us strong feeling that we are still very much a continuing part of the community, which surely is what true family practice is about."

Dr J. Reid' Practice. Successors: Dr W.R. Tough, Dr R. Steel, Dr W.G. Hardie, Dr E. Zymslowski and Dr A.K. Banerjee

We are indebted to a third year medical student, Anindo K. Banerjee, the son of Dr Banerjee of Crook, for a some extensive research into Crook history, and the history of his father's practice. He tells us that in the mid 19th century Crook was a prosperous and expanding town, and between the years 1836 and 1858 the population increased from a mere 200 to well over 4,000, and to cope with this, most of the farm land around Crook was developed into new residential areas.

The now familiar Hope Street, Gladstone Street, and Dawson Street were built and formed the commercial centre of the new town, which achieved full status as a town and parish (St. Catherine's), on 21st January, 1854. Wheatbottom was not included in the original Crook, being part of Helmington Row at that time, and a hamlet located about 2 miles south of its present position. By 1958 the present site was well developed and had acquired the name "Wheatbottom", the old site renamed "Old Wheatbottom". The original "Red House" (Dr. Banerjee's surgery), was part of that development. The first association between the house and the practice of medicine was in 1879 when Dr John Reid, M.B. a Surgeon, was the owner. He was suceeded by a Dr William Robb Tough, M.A., M.D., C.M., who held the practice until the turn of the century.

In 1905 the house and practice was bought by another Scotsman, Dr Robert Steel L.R.C.P., L.R.C.S., (Edinburgh). Two of Dr Steel's Assistants are known by name, the first a Dr Omand, who was with Dr Steel for a number of years and was well respected in the community of the time although he did not live in Red House. He was connected with Crook Town Football Club, and toured Barcelona in 1912 with the Team as a player. It is interesting to note that this connection between football in Crook and the Red House Doctors remains to this day as the present owner Dr Banerjee, is the Football Club's Doctor and organised the 1976 tour of the Club to India.

The fate of Dr Omand is however shrouded in mystery. It seems he left Crook in rather a hurry leaving behind a wife and two children and nothing was ever heard of him again.

Later Dr Steel took on another Assistant, Dr Hardie, who ultimately took over the practice. Dr Steel himself held his surgery in what is the waiting room of the present surgery, did his rounds in a motor car and even had a chauffeur. He was the only Doctor of this practice to hold public office, having been appointed Medical Officer and Public Vaccinator to the Crook Urban and Howden Districts, which gave him a place on the District Council. He also had the first telephone installed in Red House and that first telephone number, Crook 37, is still part of the number today.

Dr Steel died in 1928, his widow sold the house and practice to Dr William Graham Hardie, M.B. Ch.B (Edinburgh), who had been an assistant to Dr Steel prior to his death. He was a very popular doctor, and was responsible for the extension to Red House that is now the reception and consulting room of the surgery. Initially he did his rounds on a motor bike, but before long bought a car.

He had an Assistant called Dr Eugene Zimslowsky, popularly called Dr Eugene, who joined him after the War. He was Polish by birth but he broke away from Dr Hardie a few years later, taking a number of patients with him, to form a practice of his own in Low Mown Meadows. This was the practice eventually taken over by Dr Chesters in the other practice in Crook. Dr Hardie retired in April 1972, and was succeeded by the present incumbent Dr Arun Kumar Banerjee.

This must be the only practice in the South West Durham District that has continued in its original location, i.e. "The Red House", since it began with Dr Reid. Like all practices through its life it has seen great changes in methods of treatment used by doctors, from the "brown paper and carbolic" baby delivery kit of Dr Steel, through the methylated spirit burner for the steriliser of Dr Hardie, to electronic blood pressure and E.C.G. machines of 1988.

One cannot end the history of the medical practices in Crook without quoting from some material given to us by Dr George Pearson, which I think sums up changes which have occurred throughout the whole of the South West Durham District:

"Socially the changes in Crook District have been tremendous from the sound of pitmen's boots at all hours as they trudged to and from work, pit rows with all their doors open to neighbours, and the "dry lav." across the road, to the Council houses with all their conveniences and locked doors and lost neighbourliness."

Evenwood

Dr R.A. Milne's Practice.
Dr A. Campbell's Practice. } Successors: Dr John Neville, Dr J.R. Said.

Although it is known that Dr Sheady and Dr Hurry were in practice in Evenwood before Dr Milne and Dr Campbell it is not known when they arrived there. What is known however is that Dr Milne succeeded one of them in 1900 and Dr Campbell the other in 1908.

Dr Milne who was born in Crieff, Perthshire was brought up in Edinburgh and was a graduate of that University. Before coming to Evenwood he had been an assistant in a practice in Dawdon Colliery. At first he lived in "Brookside" later moving to his new house "Ardoch", now The Vicarage. In his early days he did his visiting rounds in Evenwood on a bicyle using his pony and trap to visit such places as Etherley, Lands, and Hamsterley. He retired to Darlington in 1947 where he died at the age of 85 in 1955.

Dr Campbell was born on Islay in the Inner Hebrides and was a graduate of Glasgow University. He had been an assistant to Dr MacKay at Crook and also in practice in Pontypridd for a short time before coming to Evenwood. When he left Crook he was presented with an illuminated address by the miners of Billy Row, Stanley and Wooley Collieries in recognition of the work he had done there. His house and surgery were in Swan Street and in his early days he did his rounds in Evenwood and the neighbouring villages, including Woodlands and Cleatlam, on his motorcycle and side-car. During the 1st World War he served in the R.A.M.C. and won the Military Cross and was mentioned in dispatches. He retired to Islay in 1947 where he died aged 82 in 1958.

It is fitting that both doctors were succeeded by some one equally respected by their patients. Dr John Neville, who took over both practices in 1947, came from Cork having qualified at the National University there. At first he practised from premises in Shirley Terrace later moving to The Vicarage but after a year or two he bought The Institute and converted it into his surgery premises. He was joined in partnership by Dr J.R. Said in 1985, and he retired two years later., Sadly he did not live long after this and he died early in 1988.

Ferryhill and Chilton

Dr Mahan' Practice. Successors: Dr M. Hunter, Dr H. Geewater and Dr R.L. Wilson

Dr L. Bruce's Practice. Successors: Dr J.B. Aitkin, Dr J. Anderson, Dr J.B. Allen, Dr O'Kane, Dr M. Stein, Dr W.T. McNeish, Dr A.B. Farmer, Dr F. Brown, Dr H. Gray, Dr R.H. Grainger, Dr H. Welsh, Dr I. Spencer, Dr N. Salfield, Dr A.J. Wright, Dr L.M.R. Hanratty, Dr A.G. Oakenful and Dr D. Sen.

In Chilton, before the 2nd World War there were two practices, one run by Dr Mahan of Killee House, Chilton, and the other by Dr Matt. Hunter at Hutton House, Chilton.

Dr Mahan was succeeded by Dr H. Geewater, who was succeeded in 1946 by Dr R.C. Wilson. Dr Wilson had Dr R.H. Grainger as an assistant in 1956-57, Dr Grainger then going to West Auckland from 1957-66 as a partner with Dr Scott and then came back to Ferryhill to join Drs Anderson, Allen and Wilson, and they later formed a group with Dr Stein in 1965. Dr Hunter was a well-known character in the Chilton area and was in practice there following the first World War, and in 1926 was Chairman of the Bishop Auckland Division of the BMA, and in the early 20's virtually at every BMA Annual Dinner he entertained with something which was entitled "The Funeral" or "A Funeral is Far Better than a Wedding". Whether this was a monologue or song we are not quite sure. His death is reported in the BMA Minutes of 19th January, 1948, and the Chairman reported his death stating "he was an old and highly esteemed Member of the British Medical Association who had rendered long and valuable service as Chairman of the Local Medical War Committee".

The practices in Ferryhill were quite different from those of Chilton, in so far as the Ferryhill doctors seemed to keep to well defined local areas and did not take patients outside their area which is more or less the pattern still followed by the group practice body today.

Practising in Ferryhill Station about the mid thirties, there was a Dr L. Bruce, practising from Eldon Terrace, and a Dr J.B. Aitkin. Dr Bruce was succeeded in 1939 by Dr John Anderson, who on the death of Dr Aitkin in 1944, took over his practice. Dr Anderson was joined by Dr J.L. Allen in 1946, and then in about 1960 they amalgamated with Dr R.C. Wilson of Chilton. They were joined by Dr M. Stein, as we have previously reported in 1965, and they all practised from 35 Market Street, Ferryhill.

In Ferryhill itself around about 1920 there were two practices, one a Dr Farmer who practised from the Manor House, and a Dr O'Kane practising from Hillcrest. Dr Farmer was a very active Member of the British Medical Association and was Chairman of the Bishop Auckland Division in 1923 and 1924.

In 1924 Dr Farmer was succeeded by Dr Fred Brown, who was later joined by a Dr H. Gray. Meanwhile,in the 1930's Dr O'Kane was succeeded by Dr M. Stein, who was joined by a Dr McNeish. In 1960 Dr Brown retired and Dr Gray and Dr Stein joined forces and they built a surgery at 35 Market Street, Ferryhill.

In 1965 Dr Gray left Ferryhill, as did Dr McNeish, and Dr Stein then joined Drs Anderson, Allen and Wilson practising in Ferryhill and Chilton. In 1966 they were joined by Dr R.H. Grainger who had come back from West Auckland. In 1967 Dr Wilson retired through illness and the practice was joined by Dr H. Welsh.

In 1967 this practice increased to six partners with the addition of Dr Spencer. In 1980 Dr Anderson and then Dr Allen retired, and they were replaced by Dr N. Salfield and Dr A.J. Wright. In 1982 Dr Salfield left and went abroad and Dr C.M.R. Hanratty replaced him. By 1987 the practice increased to seven partners by recruiting a Dr A.G.P. Oakenful, and plans for a move from 35 Market Place to much larger new premises were started. This new partner together with changes in Spennymoor, had the desired effect of removing the Spennymoor and Ferryhill area from being one of the last designated areas in the country.

In November, 1987, Dr Welsh retired through ill health and Dr D. Sen joined the practice. This year has seen Dr Taylor's premature retirement due to ill health.

As 35 Market Place was originally built for two doctors and has been extended over the years to its limits, and has been grossly overcrowded for some years, 8th October, 1988, sees the official opening of new surgery premises in Durham Road, Ferryhill.

And so we see in Chilton and Ferryhill the same sort of transition that has occurred in other areas. In other words, where there were formerly six practices there is now one. Although the patients are free to visit the surgeries and see any doctor of their choice, so far as visiting goes the doctors keep to a limited prescribed "area" for visiting purposes.

Fishburn

Dr R.J. Harbinson's Practice. Successors: Dr Robert Harbinson, Dr Ray Harbinson, Dr K. Beveridge, Dr Turnbull, Dr E. Pugh, Dr P.A. Roberts, Dr G. Johnston, Dr P.R.M. Jones, and Dr P.D. McGuiness.

The present partnership: Dr K. Beveridge, Dr E. Sutherland, Dr P.R.M. Jones, Dr P.D. McGuiness and Dr J.K. Larcombe

As we come to the far north east corner of our Health District, at Fishburn we find an interesting generation of doctors. There were no doctor practising in Fishburn until 1911 when Dr Robert James Harbinson, a graduate of Glasgow University, set up practice in the same year as the Pit was opened. He ran his surgery in Fishburn with a call house at East End, Sedgefield, until his death in 1939. Three of his sons qualified as doctors, and he was succeeded by Dr Bobby Harbinson, who unfortunately died suddenly in 1943. The youngest son, Dr Ray Harbinson, was at that time serving in the RAF, but was allowed to leave the service to run the practice. Dr Harbinson ran the practice with the aid of assistants until 1959, when he was joined by Dr Keith Beveridge and they opened a surgery in West End, Sedgefield in 1960, in addition to the original surgery at Fallscroft, Fishburn.

Dr Ray Harbinson died in 1978 and Dr Beveridge continued in practice, first in partnership with a Dr Turnbull, then in 1979, a third partner, a Dr Pugh joined. From 1980 to 1982 Drs Beveridge and Pugh continued together and then were joined by Dr Roberts. In August 1983 Dr Pugh left the practice and a Dr Johnson joined the partnership.

In February 1984 Dr Roberts left the partnership and Dr Jones joined with Dr Beveridge and Dr Johnson. In 1986 the practice became Drs Beveridge, Jones and McGuiness, and in August, 1987 a further partner, Dr Larcombe joined the practice, the partnership having amalgamated a short while earlier with Drs Fuller and Sutherland of Sedgefield, with Dr Fuller retiring shortly after that. They now have a new purpose-built surgery in Sedgefield, which was opened in 1987 and called "Harbinson House", in memory of the father and two sons who gave 65 years continuous care and attention to the people of Fishburn and neighbouring Sedgefield.

Newton Aycliffe

Original Doctors: Dr Gale, Dr V. Parker and Dr Wilson.

Successors to Dr Gale. Dr Philipson (later became Dr Gilbert), Dr G.S. Cowin, Dr D.S. Haw, Dr W.E. Chamberlain, Dr D. Morrell, Dr F.C. Saunders, Dr J.B. Jones, Dr D. Tregoning, Dr C.M. Pleasance, Dr G. Ferguson, Dr A. Gash, Dr P.D. Ramsay, Dr M. Jones, and Dr M. Howarth.

Successors to Drs Parker and Wilson: Dr Hutchinson, Dr King, Dr Smith, Dr Alcock, Dr Simhan, Dr Martin, Dr Garnham, Dr Sheldon and Dr Owen.

Newton Aycliffe of course has a comparatively recent history. It was designated in 1947 as a small new town of some 10,000 population to serve the needs of the Aycliffe Industrial Estate which was adjacent to the new town and had formerly been a war time munitions factory. It has of course greatly increased in size since then, and now has a population of around 40,000. As population moved into the new town in 1948 from the surrounding areas they were followed by their general practitioners, namely Dr Parker from Aycliffe Village, Dr Gale from Heighington and Dr Wilson from Chilton. Dr Gale and Dr Parker formed some form of partnership with each other, but when the National Health Service started they continued their partnership in Newton Aycliffe, and this partnership is recorded with the Durham Family Practitioner Committee as being on 5th July 1948 when a purpose built surgery was built there. Some time after this Dr Philipson, (who later became Dr Gilbert on marriage) came to work as an assistant. Eventually the partnership between the two seniors was dissolved and Drs Gale and Philipson went into partnership. In 1955 Dr Cowin came to work in the practice, originally as assistant, and then in 1957 when Dr Gilbert left the practice he became a partner. One interesting facet of medical practice in Newton Aycliffe in the early days was that the doctors did not see any elderly patients, and did not see any medicine relating to the ageing population. One presumes that one of the reasons for the youthful population of Aycliffe in its early days was the number of young people recently married or getting married and were looking for housing and it was readily available in Newton Aycliffe. In 1957 after the departure of Dr Gilbert, Dr Burt Chamberlain came from Bishop Auckland General Hospital and joined the practice as as assistant for approximately one year, at which time he returned to Bishop Auckland General Hospital, but is now of course senior partner in that practice. When Dr Chamberlain left Dr Haw joined the practice as an assistant and became a partner in 1959. In 1966 Dr Chamberlain returned to the practice and at this time Dr Gale was leaving and went to work for some time as an industrial medical officer at Glaxo. Shortly after this Dr Brian J. Jones who had been working in Shildon with Dr O'Neill's practice found himself alone as the O'Neills had gone to the London area to live. At the suggestion of the Newton Aycliffe practice he joined them to make up a partnership of four. In 1974 Dr David Morrell joined the practice and stayed for some three years when he returned to his fathers old practice in Chester-le-Street, and after he left Dr Frank Saunders joined the firm and is still in practice in Aycliffe. In 1982 Dr David Tregoning became a partner, but left after almost a year, we believe to return to his surgical practice in the Far East. In 1984 Dr Clive Pleasance joined the practice, but left in 1988 to return to his and his wifes native area of Liverpool. Dr Gordon Ferguson joined the practice in May, 1984, and is still a partner. Dr Amanda Gash joined on a part-time basis in 1986 and left in 1988 to work in psychiatry. In February, 1988, Dr Peter Ramsay joined the practice. On 1st May, 1988, Dr Haw, who had been in the practice in Newton Aycliffe for thirty years reached his sixtieth birthday and decided to retire. Dr Martin Jones and Dr Mary Howarth became partners in this practice in August, 1988, and Dr Brian Jones is retiring from the practice in January, 1989, when they hope to be joined by Dr Robert McKinty. This practice of Chamberlain, Jones, Ferguson, Ramsay, Martin Jones and Mary Howarth practice from their own premises at 27 Bewick Crescent, Newton Aycliffe, which of course was originated by Dr. Gale.

The Health Centre Group was originated in association between Dr Parker and Dr Kerr, (previously Dr Wilson's partner) and they formed an informal group, not financially related, but working together in 1956. This unusual arrangement continued for thirty years as others joined the group. In the 1960's Dr Hutchinson joined the group. In 1973 Dr King came to Newton Aycliffe. In 1977 Dr Smith went into partnership with Dr Hutchinson as did Dr Alcock with Dr Parker. In 1978 Dr Hutchinson died with Dr

Smith continuing the practice and in 1979 Dr Parker retired with Dr Alcock continuing in practice. In 1980 the Durham Family Practitioner Committee decided that Newton Aycliffe needed an extra doctor and created a single handed practice vacancy. This was advertised and finally a Dr Simhan was appointed, giving him an initial practice allowance which of course he would receive for three years. This initial practice allowance is given by the government whilst the doctor is collecting a list of patients. Dr Simhan did not really collect enough patients to make the practice viable and unfortunately ill health overtook him and he retired in 1984, but was not replaced. Dr King retired in 1981 and was succeeded by a Dr Martin who had held a short service commission in the Royal Army Medical Corp and was stationed at Catterick. He renewed acquaintance with two other Newton Aycliffe doctors who had also held short service commissions in the Royal Army Medical Corp namely Dr Smith and Dr Alcock. In 1986 Drs Kerr and Martin became partners and had a new junior partner one Dr Garnham. Meanwhile in 1987 Dr Kerr retired and was succeeded by Dr Sheldon, whilst in 1988 Dr Garnham moved away from the practice and was succeeded by Dr Owen.

Sedgefield

Dr Sheraton' Practice. Successors: Dr T. Thompson, Dr Hunton, Dr Bazar, Dr Hindhaugh, Dr I. Fuller and Dr E. Sutherland.

The present partnership: Dr K. Beveridge, Dr E. Sutherland, Dr P.R.M. Jones, Dr. P.D. McGuiness and Dr J.R. Lancombe.

According to information from Dr Sutherland the first doctor we know of was George Robert Sheraton. He was a distant relative of Sheraton the furniture maker and there are tales of beautiful furniture in his possession. He started practice in Sedgefield in 1860 and continued until his death in 1909. He arrived as a bachelor but soon married a local girl and they lived in Lambton House next to Eric Richards shop.

One Thomas Thompson was also a doctor in Sedgefield at the end of the 19th century and he had two sons. Dr Thomas Thompson died aged 30 of T.B. which was not uncommon in those days. His son George was apprenticed to Dr Sheraton but eventually left the apprenticeship and became a sanitary inspector in Ferryhill.

Dr Hunton followed Dr Sheraton. He lived in "Pillarbox Hall" where the Spar grocery shop now stands. Dr Hunton was killed in 1916 and next came Dr Bazar an Austrian and a devout Catholic. At first he practiced from Dunelm, 41 West End, but around 1922 when Beech House and Connor Lodge were built he moved into Connor Lodge. This house was originally called Conora Lodge but was later altered to the mere Irish "Connor".

Dr Bazar was succeeded by Dr Hindhaugh in 1927. Dr Hindhaugh, who many people still remember, arrived as a young man and stayed until his death in 1959. He was much loved and his early death much mourned. Before the opening of the Roman Catholic Church, Mass was celebrated in the dining room at Connor Lodge.

In December 1957 Dr Fuller came as a locum to the Practice and later, of course, took over the Practice and worked for many years single handed until he was joined in partnership by Dr Elizabeth Sutherland in 1965. Like all practices it has gone through considerable modernisation and upgrading and giving the service of the 1980's, largely consequent upon the opportunities given to Doctors with the Doctor's Charter of 1965. Dr Fuller's practice is one which has been more concerned than any other in research in the South West Durham Health District and he has maintained very close links with Royal College of General Practitioners in his research work with many published papers.

The practice itself has changed its character due to a large building programme of both Council and privately owned houses in the late 1960's, which virtually doubled the size of Sedgefield and changed its character from a predominately farming and artisan community to what might now be described as surburbia in a rural setting.

Shildon

Dr H. Fielden's Practice. Successors: Dr H. Widdas, Dr P.V.Anderson, Dr F. Hutchinson, Dr J.A. Anderson, Dr R. Malcolm, Dr B. Evans, Dr S.R. Gash, Dr I. Walton, Dr Lee Karen Grimes and Dr Ann McDonald.

The practice was started by Dr Harry Fielden in the 1860's in a house in the Market Place, Shildon. In about 1878 Dr Fielden built Enfield Lodge (Enfield being an anagram of Fielden) with attached surgery premises and practised from there for many years in conjunction with his son Edward.

In 1906 Dr Hugh Widdas a bachelor, joined them as an assistant at the princely salary of four guineas per week plus board and keep. In the 1st World War he served in France and Italy in the R.A.M.C. and on his return to civilian life rejoined the practice in Shildon. Dr Fielden was about to retire and his son had left to go into general practice in Torquay whereupon Dr Hugh Widdas bought the practice and Enfield Lodge. Earlier, in 1915, P.V. (Vernie) Anderson a cousin of Hugh Widdas and still a student at the Medical School, Newcastle joined the Ambulance Corp and went out to France. Although not yet qualified he was well able to cope with surgical procedures. After a while he was recalled to England and finished his medical training and resumed service in France as a fully qualified Medical Officer in the R.A.M.C. On his return home in 1919 he joined Hugh Widdas in the Shildon practice. They were in partnership for many years but both had always felt that the ideal arrangement would be to form a group practice in Shildon by joining up with the other two practices namely those of Dr R.W. Smeddle and Dr Higgins. In proposing such a plan they were some 30 years ahead of their time and in the event Shildon had one of the first if not the first group practice in the country when the three practices linked up in 1936. Dr Smeddle retired in 1939 and his patients were taken over by Dr Anderson. Later, when war broke out Dr Higgins suddenly left Shildon for Ireland without giving his colleagues any prior indication of his intentions. Eventually he returned just as suddenly as he had departed, but his absence had placed a heavy additional burden on Dr Widdas and Dr Anderson and the concept of a group practice withered on the vine.

In the long arduous war years Drs Widdas and Anderson had the help of assistants who as was usual in these times, stayed only for a few months before being called up into H.M. Forces. In 1940 one of these assistants was Dr Frank Hutchinson who married Dr Anderson's daughter Patricia herself a doctor and when he returned in 1946 after service in the Royal Navy he became a partner in the practice.

Dr P.V. Anderson had succeeded Dr Smeddle as Medical Superintendant of the Isolation Hospital at Tindale Crescent, Bishop Auckland in 1939 which added to the practice work load of which Dr Pat Anderson took her share in the early post war years. Later after her family had grown up, she returned to the practice in charge of the ante-natal clinic and family planning clinic.

When the N.H.S. was introduced in 1948 Dr Hugh Widdas retired having been in the practice for 42 years, leaving Dr Anderson and Dr Hutchinson to carry on the practice until they were joined by Dr Anderson's son John in 1952. The three remained in partnership until Dr P.V. Anderson's death in 1958. Dr P.V. Anderson, known to all his colleagues and friends simply as Vernie, was not only an astute clinician but he had an analytical mind which enabled him to explain to his often bewildered colleagues the complexities of the N.H.S. Bill of 1946 and many other medico-political problems. This ability made him an ideal choice as secretary, chairman, or member of various committees. He was Honorary Secretary of the Bishop Auckland Division of the B.M.A. for 21 years and was Chairman of the Local Medical Committee under both the old N.H.I. and its successor the N.H.S. also for 21 years. However his services were not only sought after locally but nationally too and he was a member of a special B.M.A. Committee set up to discuss the development of a comprehensive medical service in the wake of the Beveridge Report of 1942. When the N.H.S. was introduced in 1948 Vernie Anderson was one of seven doctors in England to be appointed by Aneurin Bevan as a member of the Medical Practices Committee whose purpose was to ensure a more even distribution of general practitioners throughout the country; he remained a member of this committee right up to the time of his death. In addition to these responsibilities and those of his practice he continued his connection with Tindale Crescent Hospital.

There must be many general practitioners both locally and nationally who at one time or another received valuable advice from Vernie Anderson during the years in which he held high office in medical affairs.

Dr Richard Malcolm joined the practice in 1959 and the three partners expanded the practice accommodation and facilities at Enfield Lodge, closing down their other surgery at Redworth Road. They were joined by Dr Evans in 1978 and by Dr Gash in 1982 when Dr Hutchinson retired. When Dr Evans left to take up another branch of medical practice in 1984 Dr Walton joined the practice.

Dr Malcolm retired in 1987 and was replaced by Dr Lee Karen Grimes. In the same year the surgery was moved from Enfield Lodge to purpose build accommodation in Cheapside. When Dr John Anderson retired in 1988 to be replaced by Dr Ann McDonald a family link begun by Hugh Widdas in 1906 was broken for the first time.

Shildon

Dr A.B. McA. Lang's Practice. Successors: Dr T. Higgins, Dr A.J. Smyth, Dr M.F. O'Neill, Dr D. O'Neill, Dr J.B. Jones, Dr L.G. Velangi, Dr A.K. Bhagat.

Little is known about Dr Lang who preceeded Dr Higgins in the practice and who in turn was succeeded by Dr A.J. Smyth in 1946. In 1959 Dr Mark O'Neill joined Dr Smyth in partnership and when the latter returned to Ireland in 1961 Dr Daphne O'Neill joined her husband in the practice to be followed shortly by another partner Dr J.B. Jones. The surgery accommodation was in Shildon House, Main Street. In 1967 Drs Mark and Daphne O'Neill left Shildon to go into general practice in Wimbledon and Dr Jones who was already living in Newton Aycliffe joined Drs Cowin, Haw and Chamberlain in practice there.

Drs Mark and Daphne O'Neill look back on their association with the people of Shildon with affection and with admiration for their community spirit, something not quite as much in evidence in the more affluent South.

Dr Velangi was appointed to the practice in 1967 and he was the only principal for a number of years until Dr Kagal became his partner. The surgery accommodation continued to be in Shildon House, Main Street, but as the practice expanded so did the number of staff required to cope with the work. As a result Dr Velangi and his partner Dr Bhagat, who had replaced Dr Kagal, moved to purpose built accommodation in Civic Centre Place, Shildon in 1980, retaining their branch surgery in Newton Aycliffe.

Dr R.W. Smeddle's Practice.

It is known that Dr Smeddle was practising in Shildon in 1904 but it is almost certain that he was there well before that date. He lived in Napier House at the junction of Byerley Road and Middleton Road. His surgery was just behind the house but connected to it, and was functional rather than commodious; a single room serving as a waiting and a consulting room. For many years Dr Smeddle, often clad in kneebreeches, did his rounds on foot or on a bicycle. In addition to his practice duties he was Medical Officer to Tindale Crescent Isolation Hospital.

Joe Murphy (q.v.) was his dispenser and at one time Dr Higgins, who later took over Dr Lang's practice, was his assistant. He retired in 1939 and his practice was amalgamated with that of Drs Widdas and Anderson

Spennymoor

Dr A.C. Farquharson's Practice. Partner and Successors: Dr S.V. Tinsley, Dr J.C. Livingstone, Dr R.P. Graham, Dr D. Hobbs.

Dr Farquharson left Bishop Auckland to practice medicine in Spennymoor in 1913 where his surgery accommodation was at his house, Hillingdon House. Until the early 1920's he was in partnership with Dr S.V. Tinsley (q.v.). After the 1st World War he embarked on an additional career in politics and was Coalition-Liberal Member of Parliament for the North Leeds constituency in Lloyd George's Government of 1918-22. It seems unlikely that he could combine his duties as a Member of Parliament with those of a general practitioner in a town 250 miles away without the help of his deputy in the practice and a satisfactory "pairing" arrangement in the House of Commons. His partnership with Dr Tinsley was dissolved in the early twenties but he continued to practice in Spennymoor and had a branch surgery in Byers Green where his assistant Dr Johar lived in The Hall. In addition to his short political career he was a barrister-at-law (although it seems unlikely that he practised as such) and he was prominent in B.M.A. affairs being at one time President of the North of England Branch. He retired in 1936 to be succeeded by Dr J.C. Livingstone whose surgery was at 7 Whitworth Terrace from where he conducted his practice until his un-timely death in 1942 when Dr R.P. Graham bought the practice.

In 1946 when Dr J.T. Roberts came to Spennymoor to succeed Dr Pattullo, Dr Graham moved into surgery accommodation in the practice premises owned by Dr Roberts at No. 25, King Street. Although he worked in close co-operation with Dr Roberts the two practices retained their individual identities until 1960 when they became partners. Dr Richard Graham left Spennymoor in 1966 to take up an appointment as a Regional Medical Officer in Sutton Coldfield where he is now retired. Prior to his departure he had been joined by Dr David Hobbs.

Spennymoor

Dr William Pattullo's Practice. Successors: Dr J.T. Roberts, Dr D. Miller, Dr G. Adan, Dr F.B. Kotwall, Dr A. Sanderson, Dr J.W. Chaters, Dr A.E. Sensier, Dr N. Ibbott, Dr A.J. Long.

Dr Pattulo who was a general practitioner in Spennymoor for many years lived in Tudhoe Park House fairly close to his surgery premises in 29 Kings Street. One of his assistants was Dr Janet Pope who was with the practice from 1937 to 1943 (see Part 1); she followed Dr Bulmer who had left to take over a practice of his own in Wallasey. Dr Pattullo, a conscientious practitioner and a kindly considerate employer, continued in practice until 1946 when he retired and was succeeded by Dr J.T. Roberts who was joined later in partnership by Dr D. Miller. In 1962 Dr George Adan joined Dr Roberts replacing Dr Miller and when Dr Roberts retired from the practice in 1963 the new partnership was composed of Dr Graham, Dr Hobbs and Dr Adan.

In 1970 they were joined by Dr F.B. Kotwall, Dr Hobbs having left to take up an appointment in the School Health Service. The following year the partnership moved into the new local authority Health Centre in Bishop's Place; and in 1972 Dr Andrew Sanderson joined the partnership. They continued to practise from the Health Centre until 1986 when they moved into their own purpose built accommodation in St. Andrews Road, appropriately named, Adan House, after Dr George Adan who had recently retired. That same year they were joined by Dr J.W. Charters and when he left in 1988 to take up an appointment in Community Medicine he was succeeded by Dr A.E. Sensier. Since Dr Adan's retirement Dr N. Ibbot and Dr A.J. Long have joined the practice.

Spennymoor

Dr S.V. Tinsley's Practice. Successors: Dr John Corrigan, Dr Cecilia Corrigan, Dr K.D. Wood, Dr M. Wood, Dr J.E. Staines, Dr M.S. Freeland, Dr K.A. van den Brul and Dr M.K. Flanagan.

When Dr Tinsley first came to Spennymoor in 1913 he was in partnership with Dr A.C. Farquharson. The partnership was dissolved in the early 1920's each doctor continuing in practice independently. In addition to his practice commitments Dr Tinsley was Medical Officer of Health to the Spennymoor U.D.C. He had the help of Dr Bridge-Davies as a long term assistant and also the help, for a shorter period, of Dr Francis McGuckin later to become a distinguished head of Department for Diseases of the Ear, Nose and Throat at the Royal Victoria Infirmary, Newcastle upon Tyne.

In 1943 he was joined in partnership by Dr John Corrigan whose wife Dr Cecilia joined the practice a year or two later. Dr John and Cecilia Corrigan were to be principals in the practice until they retired in 1978. The practice was conducted from surgery premises in Back Cheapside almost on the site of the present Health Centre which was opened in 1973. Both Dr John and Dr Cecilia Corrigan had quite extensive pre-general practice experience working in hospitals in a wide variety of medical posts, something which was not common in those days but which is now mandatory before entering general practice as a principal. Dr Cecilia Corrigan had been Resident Medical Officer in the Princess Mary Maternity Hospital, Newcastle upon Tyne and had a special interest in obstetrics. This stood her in good stead in the years when the vast majority of confinements took place in the home, her husband giving anaesthetics when required. In addition to his hospital posts Dr John Corrigan had obtained the Diploma of Public Health (D.P.H.) in 1940.

Like all general practitioners whose experience covers the years from the 1940's onwards they witnessed great changes in both preventative medicine and the treatment of diseases. These changes included the immunisation of children against diphtheria, whooping cough, tetanus, poliomyelitis, measles, and german measles, the virtual demise of pulmonary tuberculosis and the world wide eradication of smallpox, the introduction of a wide range of antibiotic drugs, chemotherapy for cancer, and the extension of the hospital services.

In 1963 they were joined in partnership by Dr K.D. Wood and the three continued together until 1978 when Dr John and Dr Cecilia Corrigan retired and were succeeded by Dr Wood's son Dr Michael Wood and Dr J.E. Staines. Sadly Dr Cecilia Corrigan died in 1988, a loss which was keenly felt not only by her family but by colleagues and former patients alike. Dr Wood (Senior) retired in 1981 to be succeeded by Dr M.S. Freeland and in 1966 Dr Karen van-den-Brul joined the partnership. Dr Freeland left to take up an appointment in a practice in the South of England in 1987 and the following year Dr M.K. Flanagan joined the partnership.

Spennymoor

R.S. Ross' Practice. Successors: Dr W.C. Heslop, Dr E. Brauer, Dr E.K. Hernet, Dr C.T.W. Gowdie, Dr F.B. Kotwall.

This practice had an unusual origin; Robert Stevens Ross was an unqualified practitioner almost certainly the last of his kind in the North East. He was described in the 1929 edition of Kelly's Directory of Durham as a botanical practitioner. He died in 1935 and was succeeded by Dr Heslop formerly of Bishop Auckland and Witton Park. Dr Heslop died in 1939 and was followed by Dr Ernst Brauer who had come to this country in 1934 from Breslau[2] where he had obtained the degree of Doctor of Medicine. In common with other doctors coming from Europe who wished to practise in the United Kingdom he was obliged to pass examinations for a British medical qualification. That he did so is no small tribute to his knowledge and determination.

Dr Brauer's surgery accommodation was at 23 King Street from where he ran the practice on his own until 1948 when Dr Atherton joined him as his assistant. When the latter returned to Australia in 1950 Dr E.K. Hernet took his place.

2. *Breslau was in East Germany but is now in Poland and re-named Wrocklaw.*

In 1966 when Dr Hernet left he was succeeded by Dr Gowdie but the partnership was dissolved two years later and Dr Kotwall joined Dr Brauer first as an assistant and later as a partner.

Dr Brauer left general practice in 1970 to join the School Health Service, and at about the same time Dr Kotwall joined Drs Hobbs' and Adan's practice. In 1974 Dr Brauer moved to London and continued School Health Service work there for a time later returning to general practice before finally retiring in November 1984.

Spennymoor

Dr C.T.W. Gowdie's Practice. Successor: Dr G. Adams.

When Dr Brauer's partnership with Dr Gowdie was dissolved the latter continued to practise on his own for a short time being succeeded by Dr George Adams who had previously held the senior resident post in the Princess Mary Maternity Hospital, Newcastle upon Tyne, and who had been in practice in Seahouses, Northumberland. Dr Adams practises from Spennymoor Health Centre and is one of the few remaining single handed practitioners in the County.

Tow Law

Dr J.H. Naismith's Practice. Successors: Dr R.T.E. Naismith, Dr J.J.D. Naismith, Dr R.W. Robinson, Dr A. Charlton, Dr K. Charlton, Dr I. Charlton, Dr I.C. Needham, Dr R.W. Murray, Dr J.A. Clark and Dr E.A. Finnegan.

For a considerable time prior to 1930 it was a very well known medical family, the Naismith family, who were responsible for looking after the families of Tow Law, and the surrounding districts, in an area of some 150 square miles. Dr J.H. Naismith practised in Tow Law until 1930. He had two sons who both were doctors, Dr R.T.E. Naismith and Dr J.J.D. Naismith. Dr R.T.E. (Roy) Naismith had a claim to fame, which is remembered by the older residents of Tow Law, in that he played football for Tow Law in the Northern League, and was a member of the only Tow Law team ever to win the Northern League Championship. He was in the practice for a short while before leaving to go to Slaithwaite, near Huddersfield. His son Robert who qualified as a doctor in 1944 joined his father in the Slaithwaite practice in 1947 after serving in the R.A.M.C. and later he emigrated to Canada where he was in general practice and then the public health service. He is now retired and lives in Victoria on Vancouver Island. His son Jaimie the fourth generation of doctors in the Naismith family qualified at Newcastle University and now lives in Richmond, British Columbia.

Dr J.J.D. Naismith eventually left the practice and moved to a practice in Southport. In 1930 a Dr Robinson took over the practice and in 1932 obtained an appointment at Winterton Hospital, apparently an appointment he never took up.

In 1932, the well-known man and wife team of doctors, Alfred and Kathleen Charlton, together with their four year old son Ian, moved into Grove Lodge, Tow Law. This had been the location of the practice virtually since its inception, and as was usual in those days, the surgery was attached, or within, the doctor's house. During the 1939/45 war Dr Alfred Charlton obtained an x-ray machine through the American "lease-lend" system and installed it in his surgery. He thought this would obviate his patients travelling a distance for x-rays following injuries.

According to his son, Dr Ian Charlton although he had several enquiries from the United States as to whether it was working satisfactorily he never received an account for it!

In 1951 Dr Ian Charlton qualified and joined the practice. In 1970 Drs Alfred and Kathleen Charlton retired and Dr Ian Charlton formed a medical group with numerous partners in the wide Durham area and extended the practice to the outskirts of Consett, Durham City — to Croxdale, to Brancepeth and back to the outskirts of Crook and Wolsingham, and back to Tow Law.

Dr Graham of Langley Park joined this group three years later, and they proceeded to build purpose-built surgery premises across the centre of Durham County. The practice numbers were about 25,000. However, it was interesting to note that the fringe of that practice in South West Durham, namely Tow Law, Stanley and Waterhouses area, and the outskirts of Crook and Wolsingham, retained its own little identity and eventually the old surgery at Grove Lodge was vacated and a new purpose-built surgery was opened in 1986, and the present partners in the large group who work at Tow Law are Drs Needham, Murray, Clark and Dr Ellen A. Finnegan.

And so although the Tow Law practice is now part of a ten doctor partnership it is still very much a practice on its own and has evolved like most practices in South West Durham, since the Doctors Charter of 1965, into a well organised practice giving primary medical care, with Well Woman Clinics, Baby Clinics, Hypertension, Ante-Natal and Diabetic Clinics.

There are of course, problems with Tow Law which possibly do not affect the other areas of South West Durham as much, although with improvement in roads the hazard is not as great as it used to be, namely snowfall, and there have been many occasions in the past when the districts immediately surrounding Tow Law were completely cut-off. It is interesting to note one of Dr Ian Charlton's earliest recollections when he moved from Redcar to Tow Law at the age of four to see snow drifts about six feet high in the approaches to Tow Law, something which he had never previously seen.

During the 39-45 War, Drs Alfred and Kathleen Charlton also had in their area a Maternity Home at Broomshields Hall, and these patients were later absorbed into Hardwick Hall at the end of the War, an Army Camp of about 1,000 personnel and a Prisoner of War Camp at Harperley Bank, increasing the War-time workload of the practice.

The Weardale Practices

Stanhope

Dr A. Hewitson's Practice: Successors: Dr G. Arnison, Dr C. Arnison, Dr W. Robinson, Dr J. Gray O.B.E., J.P., Dr J. O'Hara.

A strong family tradition is evident in the practice founded by Dr Andrew Hewitson at Butts House in 1823. Dr Hewitson had married Mary Arnison who was the daughter of Dr Christopher Arnison who like his father before him was in general practice in Alston. When Dr Andrew Hewitson died in 1835 the practice was taken over by Dr George Arnison a brother of his widow and on his death in 1866 he was succeeded by his younger brother Dr Charles Arnison. It is interesting to note that all these doctors qualified by apprenticeship.

In 1881 a significant event in the history of medicine in Weardale and in the County of Durham occurred when Dr William Robinson was appointed assistant to Dr Charles Arnison.

William Robinson was born in Stanhope in 1859. He had a brilliant career as a medical student and after qualifying M.B., B.S. (Dunelm) in 1881 he quickly showed his aptitude for both medicine and surgery by obtaining the additional degree of Doctor of Medicine (M.D.) and Master of Surgery (M.S.). He must have had an almost inexhaustable capacity for hard work, for in addition to being occupied by the daily demands of a busy general practice he found time to study for and pass the examination to become a Fellow of the Royal College of Surgeons. He also made a special study of the medical hazards of lead mining, pulmonary tuberculosis, and Weardale goitre, and he made contributions to medical journals about these conditions. In 1894 he moved to Sunderland where he was appointed Surgeon to the Royal Infirmary and to the Eye Infirmary in both of which hospitals he worked with distinction until he retired in 1938. Perhaps he is best remembered in Weardale as the founder of the Society for the Prevention and Cure of Consumption in the County of Durham and the founder in 1900 of Horn Hall Sanatorium at Stanhope, one of the first if not the first of its kind in the country. His achievements were recognised by the University of Durham when the honorary degree of Doctor of Surgery was conferred upon him in 1934.

Before closing this era of general practice in Stanhope mention should be made of the fact that there is a memorial in the East window of the Parish Church of St Thomas, Stanhope to George Arnison; it was presented by his brother Charles. There is a second memorial window to the memory of Charles Christopher Hewitson (son of Andrew Hewitson) who practised in

St John's Chapel. Also in the same Church is a marble tablet inscribed to the memory of Isobella Arnison wife of Christopher Arnison, Surgeon, of Allendale Town.

William Christopher Arnison who was a surgeon at the old Infirmary, Newcastle upon Tyne died in 1899, but the medical tradition of the Arnison family has been carried on in more recent times by their relatives the Hewitson family.

William A. Hewitson was a consultant surgeon at the Royal Victoria Infirmary, Newcastle upon Tyne until he retired in 1958, and his son William is at present a consultant urologist in New York.

When William Robinson departed for Sunderland in 1894 the practice was taken over by Dr John Gray who had come to Stanhope as Dr Robinson's assistant two years earlier. He moved into Butts House which was the practice headquarters until 1913 when he built "Glenroy" which was to be his new home and surgery accommodation. He was Medical Officer to Horn Hall Sanitorium, Stanhope from 1900 to 1930 and Medical Officer to the Leazes Sanitorium, Wolsingham from 1926 to 1930. Following his death in 1930 the practice and "Glenroy" were bought by Dr John O'Hara who was joined by his brother Dr Hugh O'Hara in the late 1930's. Shortly after the outbreak of the war Hugh O'Hara joined the R.A.M.C. leaving his brother John in charge of the practice with the help of an assistant, Dr Bernard.

Dr Hugh O'Hara who won the Military Cross in the Western Desert did not return to Stanhope after the war, going into general practice in Rottingdean, Sussex, later to be joined there by his brother John. In April 1948 Dr Donald Thomson and Dr Betty Thomson bought the practice from Dr John O'Hara and thus the two practices were amalgamated.

Dr Thomas Livingstone's Practice: Successors: Dr James Bannerman, Dr Donald Thomson O.B.E., J.P., and Dr Betty Thomson.

This practice was started in 1866 when Dr Livingstone, Stanhope's first University medical graduate came to live in the town. He died in 1901 and was succeeded by Dr James Bannerman a close University friend of Dr Livingstone's son. Dr Bannerman's career was interupted in 1912 by a serious motor cycle accident which left him severely disabled but from which he fought back and resumed his many duties. He had always been interested in surgery and since the nearest hospital was in Newcastle upon Tyne, quite a formidable journey in those days, his surgical skills were often in demand and Sunday mornings were set aside for his operating list. In addition to this and his other work involved in general practice he was Medical Officer of Health to the Weardale Rural District and was responsible for the care of patients in the local Isolation Hospital. In his first year as M.O.H. he had to cope with an outbreak of Small Pox which was endemic in this country in those days.

In 1938 Dr Donald Thomson joined him as his partner. Dr Thomson came from a small village near Stornaway on the Island of Lewis in the Outer Hebrides. His first language, both spoken and written, was Scots Gaelic. He was a graduate of Glasgow University and gained experience in general practice in Consett before joining Dr Bannerman. He was already on the Supplementary Army Reserve List and was called up for service in the R.A.M.C. just prior to the outbreak of war, and his place was taken almost immediately by his wife Betty who continued to work with Dr Bannerman until his retirement in 1943. There-after she ran the practice single handed until her husband's return from the war in which he had been awarded the O.B.E. for outstanding service in the Italian campaign.

In 1954 Dr Alan Liddell joined them as assistant becoming a partner in 1957. In 1961 Dr A.H. Smith who had succeeded Dr Robert Fletcher at Wearhead joined the partnership and in 1963 they opened a central surgery for Upper Weardale at St John's Chapel. In 1967 the Stanhope surgery moved from "Glenroy" to purpose built premises in Dales Street, thus ending a connection begun by Dr John Gray 54 years earlier. Later that same year Dr Smith was replaced by Dr Gelson in the partnership.

In 1970 Dr James McConchie (jun) resigned from his Wolsingham practice and moved to another practice in the south of England. Dr Gelson was appointed to succeed him thus bringing Wolsingham into the practice, and in the same year Dr J.I. Spurr was appointed as a partner. In 1971 Dr David Langford replaced Dr J.J. Gelson as a partner, the latter having emigrated to Canada. In September 1974 Dr Donald and Dr Betty Thomson retired from practice, thirty six years after they had arrived in Stanhope, where they had been senior partners together for thirty one of those years.

Dr Thomson was succeeded by Dr Peter Hill and the following year Dr Cynthia Bibby joined the partnership, and in doing so she carried on the tradition of a lady doctor in the practice which began in Dr Bannerman's time and had been continued by Dr Betty Thomson.

Dr Hill left Stanhope to continue in general practice in Newcastle upon Tyne in 1982 and was replaced by Dr J. Rutherford upon whose departure in 1985 Dr Nicholas Deytrikh joined the practice and soon became a partner. In 1988 Dr Alan Liddell retired after thirty four years in the practice at which point Dr S. Lumb who had been with the practice for a year succeeded to the vacancy.

The St John's Chapel and Wearhead Practice.

Dr Charles Christopher Hewitson's Practice: Successors: Dr A. Wood, Dr R.C. MacLennan, Dr R. Fletcher, Dr A.H. Smith.

Dr C.C. Hewitson was the son of Dr Andrew Hewitson the founder of the first general practice in Stanhope. He established the practice in St John's Chapel probably sometime between 1850 and 1860; he died in 1896 at the

shire House on the death of Dr Smith, but alas, he died not long afterwards. At that time the sole employee in the practice was a Miss Greta Baines, who was invaluable as a dispenser and secretary and loyal supporter of the doctor, and who later became a District Nurse with the Health Authority in Bishop Auckland.

Dr Claude Fenwick (formerly of Craghead) took the house and practice after the death of Dr McPherson. Dr Fenwick retired due to illness on 31st March, 1957, and died in the mid-sixties. He had as his assistant the late Dr John Neville in 1947, later of Evenwood, and his brother William (Bill) for a while in 1948, before he went to Cockfield.

Next came Dr M. Raphael, who is now in Sunderland. Drs Behan and Munroe, and finally Dr Grant Ferguson, now of Crook, from April '53 to January '54. In 1954 Dr Cedric Scott came as an assistant and then as the partner. Dr Grainger stayed from May '57 to September '66, when he moved to Ferryhill, where he is now the Senior Partner. This of course, left Dr Cedric Scott single-handed in the West Auckland practice, and at that time there was a suggestion that he join the Dr Cama practice, as Dr Leonard Cama was leaving in a year. From 1st October 1966, Drs Cama, Clark, Shuttleworth, Scott and Lewis closed the Devonshire House surgery and had a purpose-built surgery built at Manor Road, St. Helens. In May 1968 Dr C.M. Scott left the practice and became part of the Regional Medical Service under the DHSS and is still a Regional Medical Officer with that Service.

The West Auckland practice with a call house at Toft Hill, was an entirely dispensing practice until Mr John Welsh M.P.S. took over the former Drugist's shop in the village (presumably from where the infamous Mary Ann Cotton of yester-year purchased her poison). Mr Welsh later moved the Chemist's shop to St. Helen's Auckland to be nearer the new surgery. This practice has changed over the years from being semi-rural to semi-urban, now virtually urban.

Dr Scott recalls one of his most traumatic experiences was delivering an unmarried woman in the lavatory of the garage at Royal Oak and giving the infant mouth to mouth resuscitation all the way to Bishop Auckland General Hospital. He then had to go and tell a lady that she was once again a Grandmother as no one else had the courage to do so. There was also another interesting side to the practice at West Auckland, and in a way, demonstrates attitudes of different types of patients: One Sunday night Dr Grainger did not get home from his weekend off as he was travelling through a very severe snow storm. His mother-in-law telephoned Dr Scott to see if he had arrived safely but there was no news of him there or elsewhere on route. On Monday morning the practice had two calls to Bolam, one to visit at Leggs Cross Cottage, and the other to visit a house in the village "because a sick note was due and they could not get out". Dr Scott explained that he also could not get out and that Dr Grainger had not returned. Dr Grainger managed to get down by 10.00 a.m., apparently having abandoned his car at Leggs Cross. He had knocked on Leggs Cross Cottage door for shelter to be met by the inhabitant who said "I didn't expect you tonight Doctor, but in the morning after surgery"! After explanations Dr Grainger stayed the night and after evening surgery on the Monday a party was taken up to get his car out of the snow at Leggs Cross. The patient who wanted the quarterly sick note delivered came down later in the week and berated Dr Scott. She demanded to know if he had so many patients that he could not be bothered (it would have involved Dr Scott in a 9 mile return trip on foot to deliver that sick note — such is the attitude of some patients).

Willington

Dr W. Allen's Practice: Successors: Dr R.E. Brown (sen), Dr R.A. Brown (jun), Dr Alison Kirk, Dr A. McQueen, Dr R.A. Middleton, Dr B.S. Sarnaik.

This practice like several others in the S.W.D.H.A. had a strong family tradition until fairly recent times. Dr Allen was Dr R.E. Brown's stepfather and Dr R.A. Brown ("Dr Archie" as he was known to everyone) the latter's son. The practice was mainly industrial with coal mining predominating but there was also a rural component.

Dr Jean Mitchel who was an assistant to Dr Brown from 1941 to 1947 describes the practice then as being:

"Mainly composed of miners and their families with a fair sprinkling of farmers, trades people, teachers and private house holders. The practice area was quite widely scattered taking in two mining villages, Oakenshaw and Sunnybrow and a number of smaller villages and hamlets; Helmington Row, High Jobs Hill, Wheatbottom, Seldom Seen, Never Seen, Newfield, Todhills, and surrounding farms like Nutty Hag, Wether Hill, The Middles, and Stonechester.

The surgery at 96 High Street contained an extremely well equipped dispensary with a full time dispenser. There were Call Houses in Oakenshaw and Sunnybrow and a typical days work consisted of morning surgery followed by visits to Willington, and then on to Oakenshaw to pick up new visits there. When those and the follow-up visits had been done it was back to the surgery with a list of prescriptions for the dispenser to make up and have ready for the family messenger to collect. After that more visiting in Willington, a round in Sunnybrow and perhaps a visit to a farm or two and then back for evening surgery. An ordinary day began at 8.30 a.m. and ended at about 8.30 p.m."

Dr Archie Brown was the colliery surgeon and the work involved is described by Dr Mitchel in Part I. Another lady doctor, Dr Alison Kirk was an assistant in the practice from 1940 to 1941, returning in 1946 and becoming a partner in 1948. Dr A. McQueen who had acted as locum tenens for

Dr Brown in 1952 joined the practice as a partner the following year. He opened a second surgery at 31, Low Willington, the equipment and staffing of which foreshadowed today's consulting suites. Dr Brown retired in 1962 and Dr R.A. Middleton joined the practice shortly afterwards.

Dr Archie Brown was an immensely popular general practitioner and no doubt his family ties with Willington had something to do with this, but such was his ability and personality that he would have been just as popular without those family ties. He served in the R.A.M.C. in the 1st World War and was present on the first day of the Battle of the Somme on July 1st 1916. The carnage of that fearful day made a profound impression upon him and every July 1st there-after he had a few moments of silence as a mark of respect to the fallen.

In 1963 Dr McQueen left to take up a career in pathology at Glasgow University and Dr Kirk retired from general practice in December 1969 to take up work in Child Health and later in Industrial Health. She is now retired but still lives in Willington.

Dr B.S. Sarnaik joined the practice as a partner to Dr Middleton in April the following year but the partnership was dissolved just over three years later, each of the doctors continuing as single handed practitioners.

Dr Brewis' Practice: Successors: Dr A. Crichton, Dr P.J. O'Grady, Dr P.A. Middleton, Dr A.J. Eames, Dr B.S. Sarnaik, Dr M. Baker, Dr G. Wilson.

Dr Brewis was succeeded by Dr Alexander Crichton in 1946 and was joined in partnership by Dr P.J. O'Grady in 1957. There were two separate surgeries in the practice at the time, one at Dr Crichton's house "Eskdale" and another at 24 Commercial Street. When Dr Crichton died in 1974 Dr Middleton who was on his own at the time joined Dr O'Grady in partnership and their surgery accommodation was combined and moved to Albion Place.

Amongst Dr Crichton's duties was one which must have brought him considerable pleasure. He was Honorary Medical Officer to Willington Football Club and in 1950 when they reached the final of the Amateur Cup at Wembley, he was responsible for getting one of their key players fit in time for the match against their Northern League rivals Bishop Auckland. The match is remembered by followers of amateur football as one of the greatest of all time, especially by supporters of Willington who won 4-0.

In 1977 Dr A.J. Eames joined the partnership and in April that year they moved into the newly built Health Centre in Chapel Street. When Dr O'Grady retired at the end of December 1987, to be succeeded by Dr M. Baker, Dr Sarnaik whose surgery accommodation had also moved to the new Health Centre when it was opened joined the other doctors forming a single group practice. Dr Eames emigrated to New Zealand in 1988 and his place was taken by Dr G. Wilson so that the four doctor group now practice under the title of Drs Middleton, Sarnaik, Baker and Wilson.

Sir James Mackenzie

No account of general practice in South West Durham would be complete without mentioning the connection, albeit a tenuous one, with the world's first cardiologist, Sir James McKenzie.

In July 1878 the newly qualified Dr James MacKenzie came to Spennymoor to act as a locum tenens for a general practitioner there. After two or three months he moved on to take up similar duties for Dr Joseph Keay of The Red House, Crook where he stayed until November. His interest in heart disease began early in his career and after many years as a general practitioner in Burnley he was a recognized authority on this subject. By the time he was appointed to the first Department of Cardiology at The London Hospital he was nationally and internationally famous for the work he had done as a general practitioner. This included the invention of the polygraph, an instrument which recorded simultaneously the apex beat of the heart, the radial pulse, the carotid pulse, and the venous pulse, and which foreshadowed the development of instrumental investigation of the heart especially by the electrocardiograph.

He was knighted for his services to medicine in 1915 and is rightly regarded as being the world's first cariologist.

The Lighter Side of General Practice

Apart from relations and very close friends, few people enjoy the general practitioner's privilege of informal access to other people's homes. A knock on the door or a ring of the bell followed by the almost simultaneous opening of the door with the cheery shout of "Doctor!" announces the practitioner's arrival. The time of day dictates the presence or absence of other members of the family. If the children are at home it is by no means certain that the television, radio or music centre will be switched off; each is a well know juvenile tranquiliser. Dogs are sometimes an additional hazard, doctors being second only to postmen as a target. Some doctors of course, are dog lovers themselves in which case the resident dog can provide an additional bond in the doctor-patient relationship. However, the doctor less adept at doghandling can take comfort from the speed at which such news travels amongst his patients and in next to no time the dog will be safely secured on visiting days. There are other animal hazards, and unlikely as it may seen, one patient kept a ferret in his bed, giving rise to some very puzzling clinical signs when the lower abdomen was examined. A python has been sighted in one house, but thankfully confined to a cage. Budgerigars have been known to flutter about indoors; it is surpriseing how accurate their low level bombing attacks can be.

Thirty years or more ago it was not unknown in The Batts, Bishop Auckland, for goats and poultry to share the accommodation with the family. When one general practitioner was visiting a family who had been rehoused elsewhere in the town he expressed no great surprise when he met a horse coming downstairs from the bathroom.

Dr Dawes describes two incidents when visiting patients in Close House in the early 1950's. The first one concerns his partner.

"There was one occasion when Dr Oliver returned home with two large white eyes and a black face. This had been caused by visiting a patient whose standard of hygiene was not what it should be. In order to counteract this he had lit his pipe and casually put his hand on the mantlepiece when, to use his own words "the whole bloody issue fell into the place in a cloud of soot". There was nothing for him to do but return home, have a bath and resume his work".

The second concerns Dr Dawes himself when making a night-time visit: "I entered the back of a house which was pitch black, mainly because the street lights were out of action, and having hammered on the door and received no reply, decided to enter. Feeling my way through the darkened room, I suddenly pitched forward into a hip bath filled with cold, dirty water, which had been used by a miner returning from his work two hours previously".

The moral of these two stories, says Dr Dawes, is never to enter a darkened room and once in the room, never touch anything unless it is known to be securely fixed to the wall!

Surgery consultations have been known to provide a welcome light relief from time to time. An athletic young lady complaining of abdominal pain consulted her doctor who, using the English language less precisely than he might have done, said "Jump up onto the couch and I'll have a look at your tummy". To his astonishment the girl took one or two springy steps, leapt up onto the couch and looking down on him from a height of some 8 or 9 feet, asked "Are there any more tests you would like me to carry out, Doctor?".

PART IV

THE HOSPITALS OF SOUTH WEST DURHAM

by

Frank Robertson MD FRCP
Retired Consultant Physician,
Bishop Auckland General Hospital

Preface

This account of the hospitals of South West Durham has been written after consulting the records of the minutes of the committees of the various hospitals. The earlier minutes are held in the Durham County Records Office at County Hall, Durham. I am very grateful for all the courtesy and help given to me by Mr David Butler, the County Archivist and his staff over a period of six months.

Later records were held at Winterton Hospital and at the South West Durham Health Authority Headquarters at Claremont in Bishop Auckland. Mr A. Tonge brought all the Winterton volumes to Claremont and both he and Mr P. Brotherhood gave much help concerning Winterton. Although records exist in Durham since the opening of Winterton in 1858 it was soon clear that a separate book would be needed to deal with Winterton alone, accordingly I decided to commence the account only from the start of the National Health Service in 1948.

The records dealing with Horn Hall, Leazes and Holywood Hall Hospitals are all in the County Records Office and describe the start of one of the earliest hospitals altered to deal only with the widespread problems caused by tuberculosis, and then in the 1950's following the discovery of streptomycin and the drugs that were later used, the rapid decline and almost eradication of the disease so that two of the hospitals could be shut and the other, Horn Hall, used for different diseases.

Dr Hugh Bannerman, now living in Somerset kindly lent me a book of reminiscences written by Dr William Robinson, but I have not actually quoted from it.

Mr George Metcalfe and Prof D. Scott kindly read the manuscript and gave helpful advice.

The staff at Claremont provided a room in which to write and consult the records and I am grateful to Mrs Angela M. Fleming and her colleagues for their help and encouragement. Mrs Elsie Copeland cheerfully supplied me with coffee during the writing. Special thanks are due to Mrs Jean Hyslop for her typing and for accepting so pleasantly all the alterations that were inevitably required.

The comment concerning the bleak state of many poor law institutions at the start of the NHS was taken from an account of the first thirty years of the NHS published by HMSO, and I am grateful for the permission of the Controller of HMSO to do so.

Mr David M. Ryan, District General Manager and Mrs Erika R. Wallis, Chairman, of the South West Durham Health Authority gave help and encouragement.

Many other people, as they heard of the project, expressed interest, gave encouragement and recalled events. I cannot mention them all by name, but I gladly express my grateful thanks.

Dr D.T. Prescott who has had a long association with the Lady Eden Hospital and the Princes Street Maternity Home, wished to write about these two hospitals and I am grateful to him for doing so.

Conditions in Bishop Auckland in 1853 and some Infectious Diseases

Before 1890 there were only two hospitals in South West Durham. Winterton County Asylum as it was then called had been built in 1857 and the Poor Law Institution in Bishop Auckland had been in existence before 1834. In 1853 it was rebuilt and enlarged on the present site of Bishop Auckland General Hospital. In those days all small towns were required by law to provide accommodation for the destitute. These, usually men, wandered from village to village doing a little work en route, could be given a night's lodging, and in return did some work in the institution before setting off on the road again. The men were expected to break stones, do gardening or labouring tasks, and the women to clean, or assist in the kitchen or laundry. Hence the institution was usually referred to as the workhouse.

Some of the inmates — as they were called — were old and infirm, others ill, and hence sick and infirm wards had to be made for them. In addition the destitute ill people in the community could be committed by the Relieving Officer and the District Medical Officer to the Institution for care, treatment or to die. Unmarried girls who were pregnant were admitted for delivery and a nursery had to be provided. Children who were ill, neglected, or abandoned by their parents were taken in. If a wife was deserted by her husband she and her children could be admitted. Mentally defective people who couldn't be cared for in the community could also be taken in and before Winterton was completed there were some adult psychiatric patients. The demand for nursing care was thus always present. However, nursing as we know it was in its infancy and trained nurses quite rare.

It is difficult to imagine the conditions of life in the middle of the last century yet we need to know something about it in order to see how the hospitals came to be built and the standards required, not according to modern day views but to fit the conditions, needs and knowledge of those times.

In 1853 an enquiry was carried out by Thomas Webster Rammell who came to Bishop Auckland in response to a petition by more than one tenth of the ratepayers of Newgate, the Borough, and Bondgate which together made up the township of Bishop Auckland. Mr Remmell was the Superintendent Inspector sent by the General Board of Health in London to see what was needed to bring into force the new Health of Towns Act. I have extracted some details from the enquiry from Fordyce's History of Durham published in 1855 and from the Minutes of the Local Board of Health.

Mr Rammell held the enquiry in Shepherds Inn in Bishop Auckland. The Curate of Bishop Auckland, two Solicitors, a Surgeon, the Secretary to the Bishop of Durham, a Land Surveyor, an Architect, the Registrar of Births, and the Relieving Officer together with four other men were present.

The mortality rate was 28.6 per thousand much of it due to infective diseases. Nearly half — actually 43%, of the deaths were in children under the age of five years.

The main industries were the collieries and iron works which were daily increasing. The Bishop Auckland and Weardale railway had been completed in 1840.

One turnpike road was called Bowes to Sunderland Bridge turnpike road and passed through the town by Newgate Street and Gib Chare.

The town was lighted by gas provided by a joint stock registered company. The gas works opened in 1835 near the railway station. There were between fifty and sixty street lamps but the newer areas of town — South Terrace, Tenters Street and Etherley Lane did not have a gas supply.

There were probably not more than a dozen water closets in the town. Most of the respectable houses had privies communicating with covered cesspools. In lesser houses, one or two privies were allocated in common to all the houses in a court or alley, mostly with open cesspits behind them. These also received household slops, ashes and vegetable refuse. Sometimes the cesspits discharged liquid into the drains. At the south end of Newgate Street, one privy served forty persons and in Etherley Lane another was also used by forty people.

The Curate complained that "a tannery at the bottom of Wear Chare is a great nuisance and a north wind blows the stench all over the town. Likewise a tallow manufactory in Back Bondgate causes great nuisance". There were about six slaughter houses in the centre of the town. The offal was kept in pits until they were full. Blood was usually thrown onto a dung heap. In one case it was washed into a sewer.

Most drains were open and led nowhere. Some were level e.g. in Fore Bondgate. The smell was intolerable before stink traps were put in. When last opened the drains were filthy and in some places had one and half feet of deposit. A man slipped and nearly suffocated in it.

Water was obtained from wells in some private premises, or from a few natural springs — the chief being at the end of Newgate Street and also by a pipe carrying surplus water from a cistern in the Castle Yard to the PANT in the Market Place. The better class house caught roof water for washing. The chief requirement in the area was for more water. The water was analysed from the wells and springs and except for that from the River Wear was regarded as fit to be recommended for the town water supply.

Dwellings — Taking in lodgers prevailed especially in Irish households. In Irish cottages a single family rarely occupied more than one room. Indeed three or four families sometimes used one room, without bed, chair or table. A few stones were put in a circle round the fire for seats and straw or shavings served to lie upon. The Irish Quarters were in Back Bondgate, Townhead and Newgate, being principally back yards. The English labourers in collieries lived in better cottages but still only had parts of a house for the family. Their houses were generally decently furnished and many were very clean.

Lodging houses were all unregistered. There were twenty nine in all. Of these, only three could be considered at all decent. They charged 2d or 3d per night and one of the better contracted with the unions (i.e. the "work-house") to receive lodgers who could not be admitted to the workhouse and these provided night accommodation for the casual poor. This, said the report, prompted vagabondage and immorality.

The Police Superintendent reported on a house kept by Nathan Green. There were 10 rooms, the largest of 18 feet by 15 feet by 6 feet high. In all there were 22 beds but when the Superintendent visited at night there were 35 to 45 inmates. In one room he counted 17 men, women and children all sleeping together. This was one of the best kept lodging houses. The lodgers slept naked, this was thought to lessen the risk of contracting infectious diseases and vermin in the clothes.

In Townhead there were 130 inhabitants in 37 rooms and in Back Bondgate 156 inhabitants in 29 rooms.

In 1853 there were three or four cases of cholera and odd cases of typhus fever.

Mr Rammell recommended that the Public Health Act should be applied to the township. Drainage of the substratum of the town and an efficient surface and refuse drainage should be carried out. There should be a plentiful supply of pure water and adequate privy accommodation in connection with the efficient drainage and water supply. He also said that there should be improvement in the road ways and the removal of many offensive nuisances. Also needed was improvement of the dwellings of working classes and regulations to prevent overcrowding in these and also of the common lodging houses.

Such was life in the town in 1853. By 1950 there were still numerous houses without water closets. The tannery mentioned in the report was for the day. Those above the age of 60 had tea or coffee allowed.

The new building was overcrowded by 1863 and a further 50 places had to be provided by raising the height of the front building to provide more sleeping accommodation, and in view of the extra work the salary of Dr Hutchinson, the Medical Officer was raised to £30 a year.

By 1892 Dr Mark Wardle had become Medical Officer to the Institution. I do not know the date of his appointment or whether he immediately followed Dr Hutchinson.

Like many other doctors Dr Mark Wardle did some surgery and in 1892 he removed a cataract from a woman patient. I think this was done in the home of the patient. She was so pleased that she invited a friend also suffering from a cataract, to consult Dr Wardle. He then presented a bill to the Guardians for five guineas for each operation.

He also operated on a baby of 19 months and removed a pin from the abdomen. I am grateful to Mrs Mary Mawby, grand-daughter of Dr Mark Wardle for letting me see a book of cuttings which included a copy of the account of this baby written by Dr M. Wardle in the Newcastle and Durham Medical Journal. Thc baby was about 12 months old and ran across the floor with a hatpin in his mouth, the point was upwards, the pin with a glass head at the end was about six inches long. The child fell and the mother declared the pin was swallowed. After anaesthetising the child with chloroform Dr Wardle found nothing and concluded the pin was lost, not swallowed. He thought the length of the steel pin and its inflexibility made swallowing unlikely. However, over the next few months the child would not lie down and sat curled up in a little rocking chair, getting steadily into a weak and emaciated condition. Some months after the occurrence an abscess the size of a walnut appeared in the abdominal wall. Under anaesthetic he opened the abscess and then the abdominal cavity when he found four inches of the steel pin, much eroded. He thought the bead and remaining two inches had entered the gut, and been passed unnoticed. The pin had entered the stomach and then perforated the wall and caused the abscess. The wound healed by first intention and on calling on the fourth day he says he found the mother out and the child playing on the floor. He asked for 50 guineas from the Guardians for this. The committee considered this request for a long time and then said that as a District Medical Officer he already received a salary (around £30 a year) for his duties no payment was justified. They were prepared however, to offer him a gratuity of five guineas for the child and three guineas for each of the two cataract patients as an acknowledgement of his skill and attention in these cases. It was common practice for the Guardians all over the country to award extra payments to their Medical Officers for special work, although as recipients of a fixed salary they could be required to carry out all normal work. They also provided the necessary drugs for the one salary. As a result of the Bishop Auckland Guardians reluctance to pay the extra honorarium the British Medical Journal mentioned this and suggested that the doctors might feel it unwise to seek a post with that authority.

Next year 1893 Dr Wardle performed two more cataract operations but the committee refused to pay until the Relieving Officer reported on the condition of the patients. When he issued a favourable report the committee decided that he must make a further report in a months time and it was only after three reports had been received that they paid ten guineas for the two cases. They also set up a committee to consider future surgery. I suspect they could see their funds disappearing fairly rapidly. The committee decided that no further gratuities would be paid unless the committee itself had given consent to the operation. After protests by Dr Wardle that delay in receiving permission might endanger lives, they agreed that permission from the clerk would suffice in urgent cases.

There had been a nurse in the sick wards of the institution but she had resigned, and in March, 1891 the local government board inspector said that a replacement had not been appointed. The local government board also said that the Guardians must give the matter urgent attention but the Guardians resolved to stick to their previous decision not to consider an appointment until the chronic ward was opened "so that medicines could be dipensed by someone who could read". I think that up to 1893, various staff members had been given the duty of looking after the sick and given the temporary title of nurse, or else other inmates had done the work. In the year 1894 however, the committee at last agreed to appoint one nurse whose sole responsibility would be the care of the sick and infirm. She was to be a certificated nurse and the committee drew up rules.
"The nurse would record the temperature of the ward morning and evening and put the figure in her report book.

She would take care that no improper words or indecorous actions, are at any time permitted, or that any immoral books, songs or printed matter are introduced into the wards.

Apart from visiting days no unauthorised person shall have communication with the patient".

Rules were also laid down concerning the opening of windows. The windows were to be opened at 7 a.m. from 26th March until 29th September and at 8.30 a.m. on the remaining days of the year. There were rules about washing of clothes, changing bed linen and the care of bathrooms and toilets.

The nurse would have three hours off duty twice a week and return to the infirmary not later than 10 p.m. She could take three hours off on alternate Sundays for divine worship. There was to be 14 days holiday a year.

The rules went on to say that "friends visiting the nurse must obtain permission from the Master and if such permission was granted the visitor must not stay more than one hour and it was to be distinctly understood that only two visitors per week would be allowed".

The salary was £30 per year.

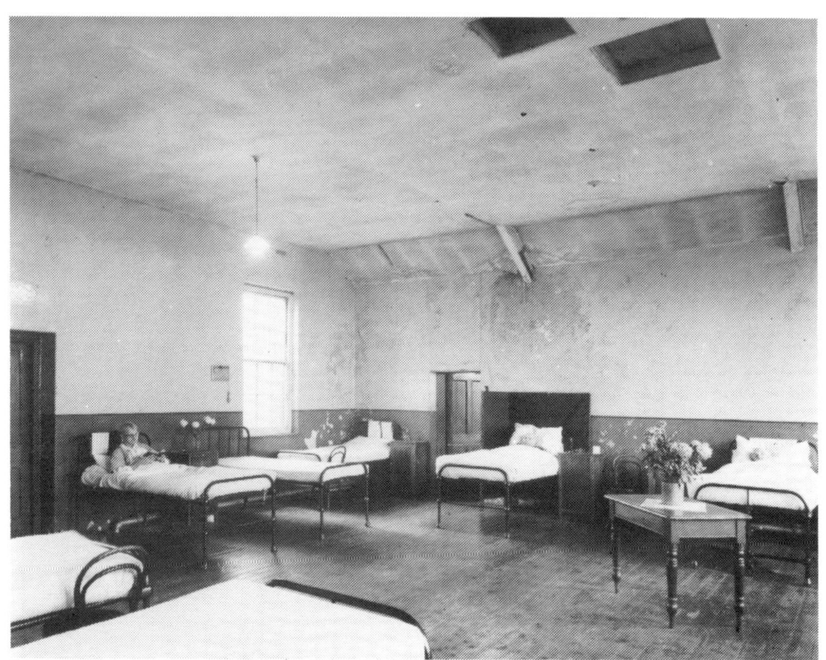

A ward in Block 3 in Bishop Auckland General Hospital, about 1948.

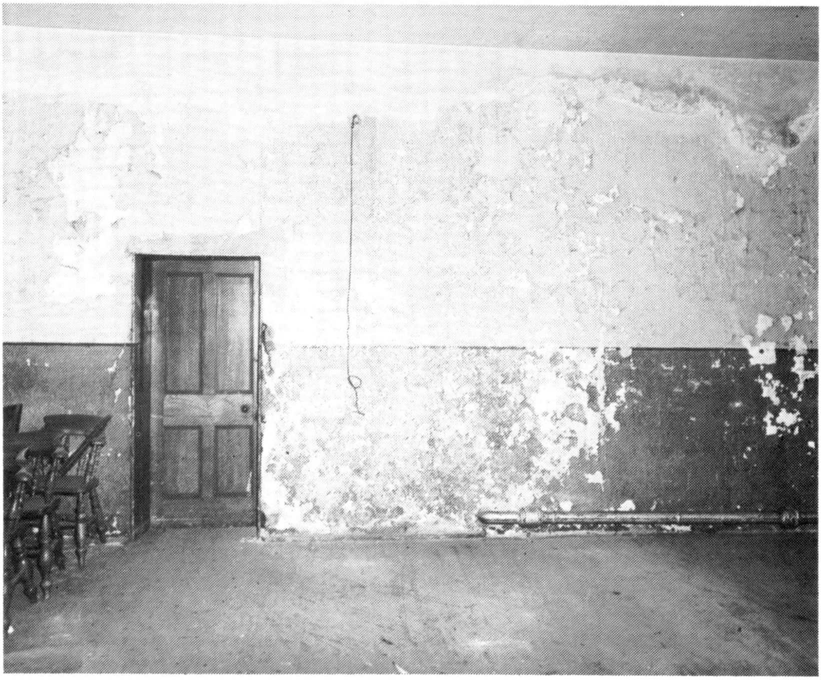

A ward in Block 3 immediately after closure.

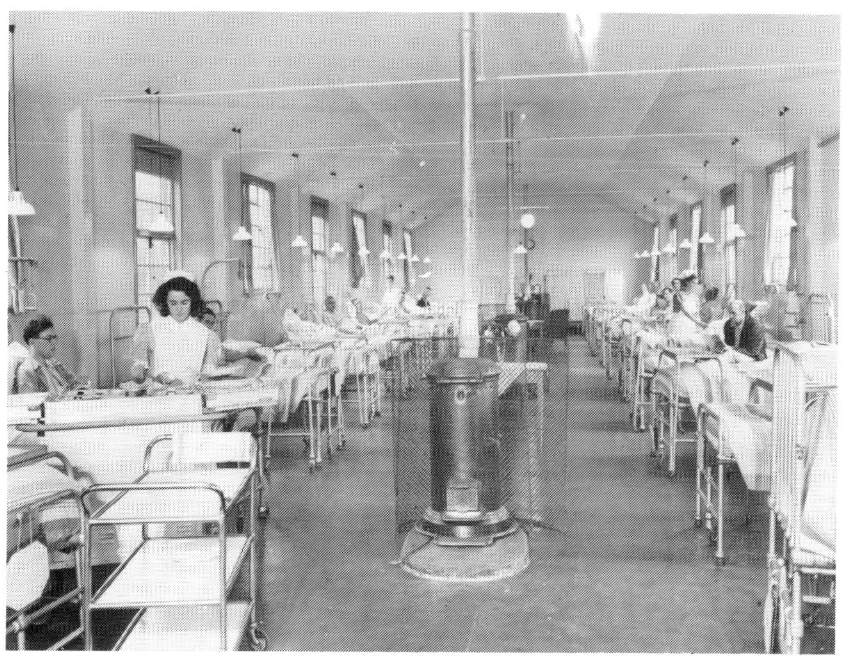

A ward in Bishop Auckland General Hospital in the 1950's. Note the coke stove.

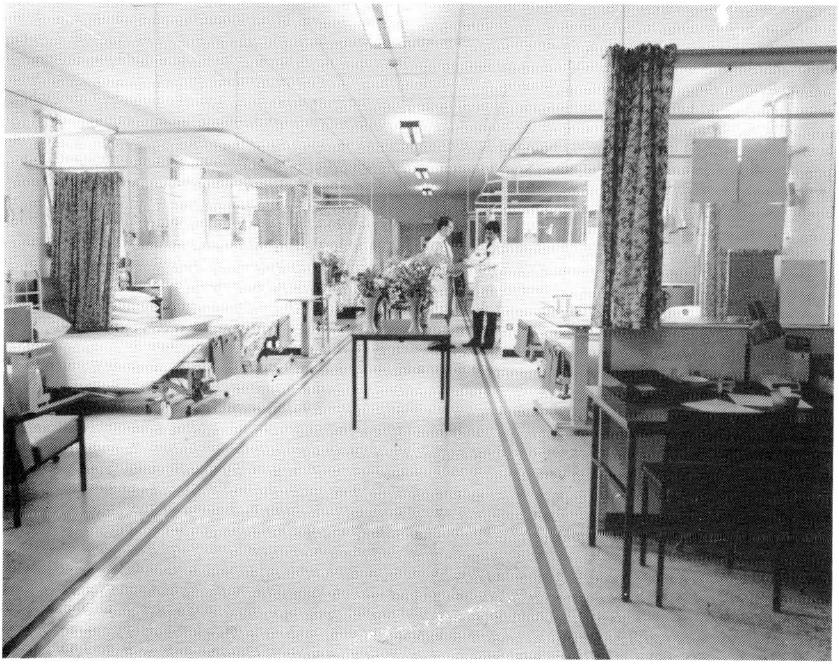

The same ward in 1989.

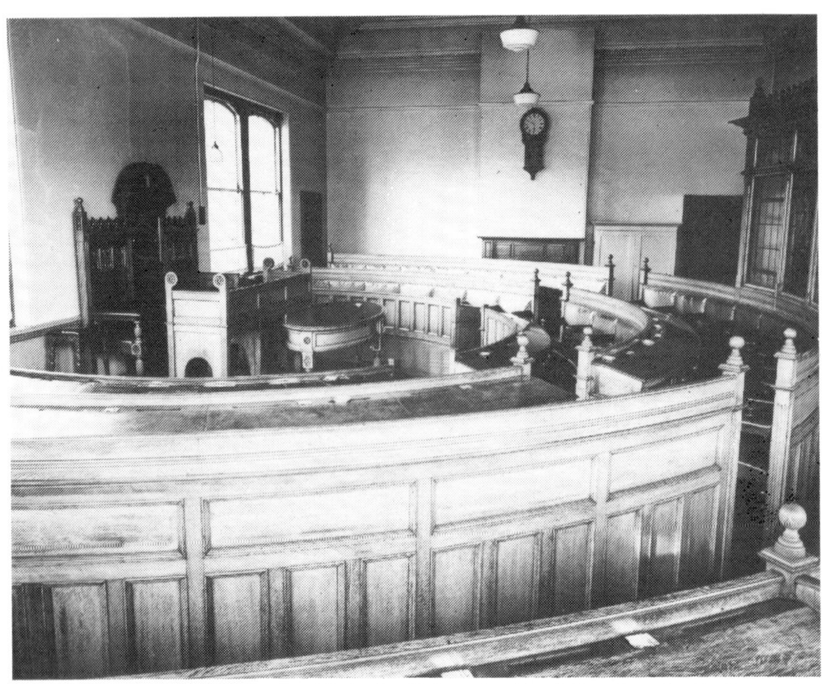

The Board Room which served both the Bishop Auckland Poor Law Institution and later The Bishop Auckland General Hospital.

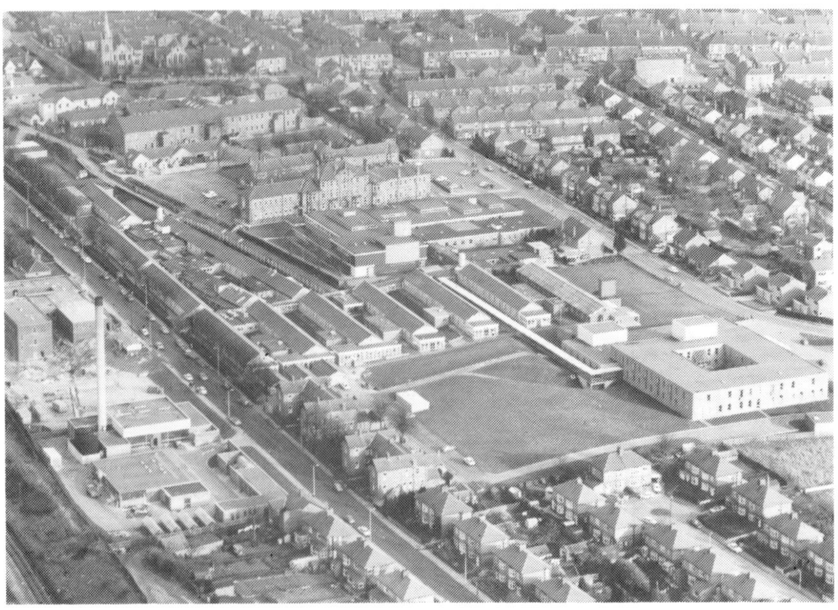

Aerial view of Bishop Auckland General Hospital, 1977.

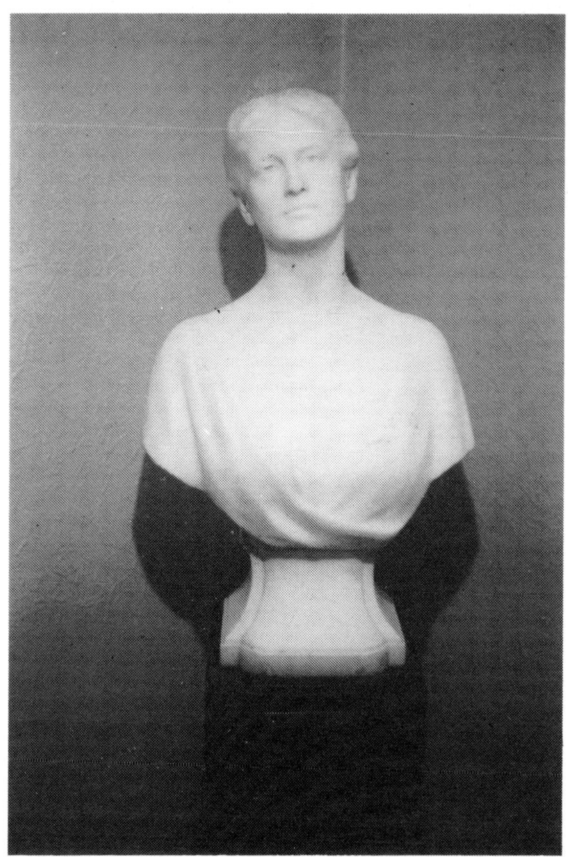

Bust of Lady Sybil Eden presented to the Lady Eden Hospital
by Sir Timothy Eden and family.

SICK & YE COMFORTED
LADY EDEN
Souvenir
of the opening of
COTTAGE HOSPITAL
by
The Auckland
Times & Herald.

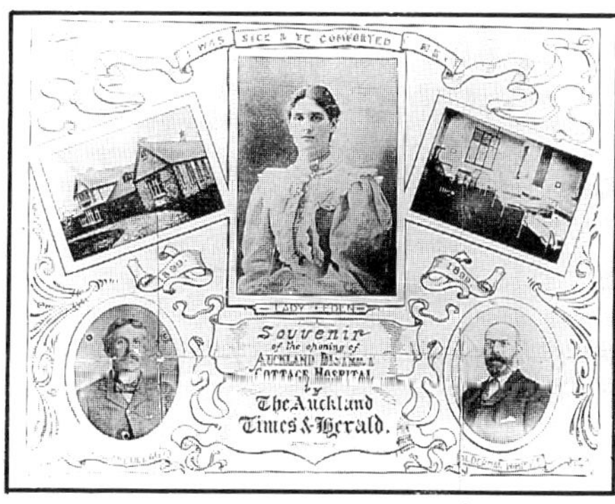

A souvenir of the opening of the Auckland District Cottage Hospital, 1899.
Later re-named The Lady Eden Cottage Hospital.

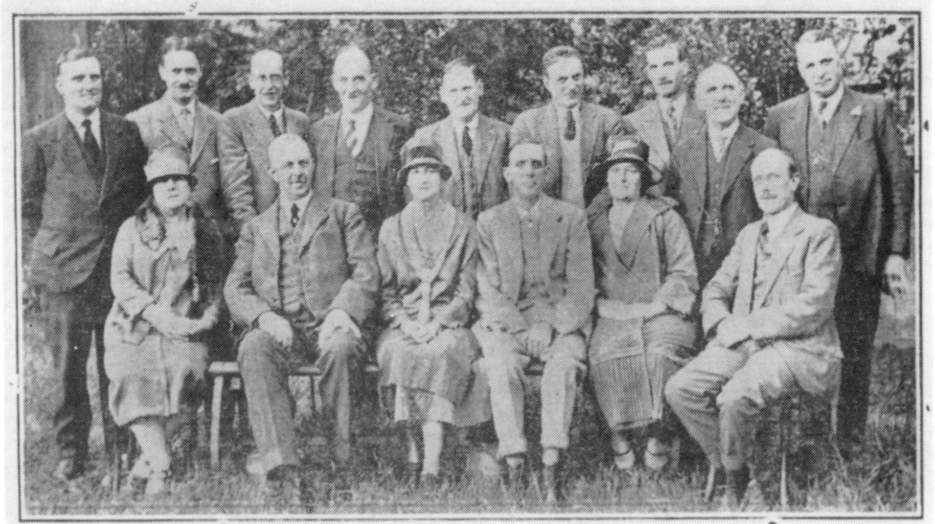

Left to right: Mr. W. Kennair (Sec.) Mr. Hirst, Mr. E. Abbey Coun. Matt 'C. Robson, Mr. E. Donn, Mr. G. Somervell, Coun. C. Gent, Mr. Thompson Mr. Hull; Mrs Firby, Supt. Headen (Marshall), Sybil Lady Eden Coun. G. C. Young (President), Coun. Mrs. Bull, Mr. G. W. Rudd (Vice-President)
Photo and Blocks by " Auckland and County Chronicle"

Committee of Lady Eden Cottage Hospital, 1927.

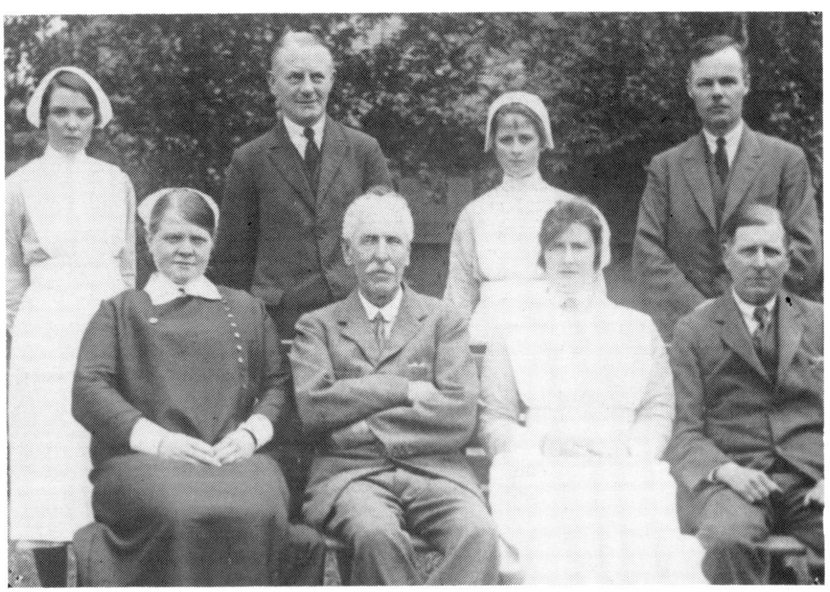

The staff of The Lady Eden Cottage Hospital, 1926.

Back Row L to R:-
Nurse Hallam, Dr T.E. Ferguson, Nurse Knaggs, Dr V.H. Wardle.
Front Row L to R:
Matron Melling, Dr T.A. McCullagh, Staff Nurse Jones, Dr A.C.H. McCullagh.

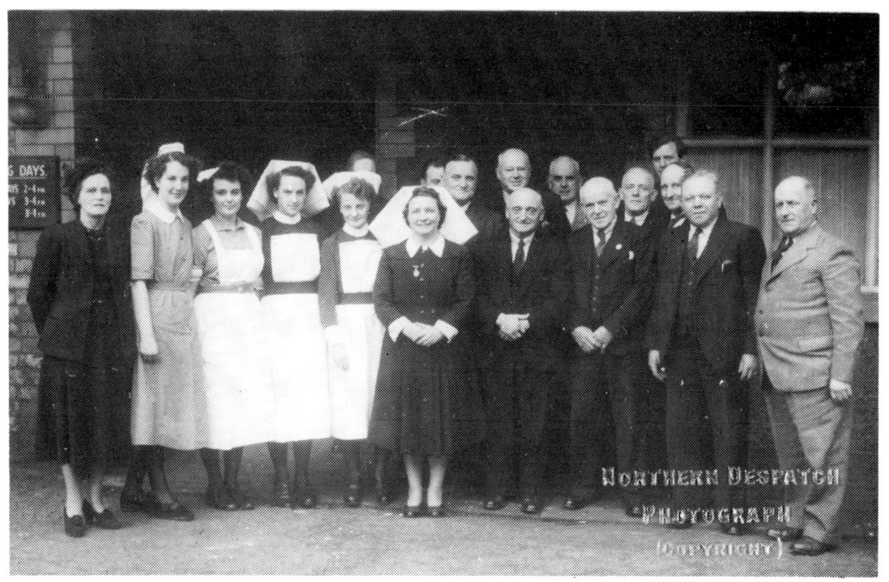

Some members of the S.W. Durham Hospital Management Committee with Matron Dinning, Sister Snailham and Nursing Staff of the Lady Eden Hospital, 1950.

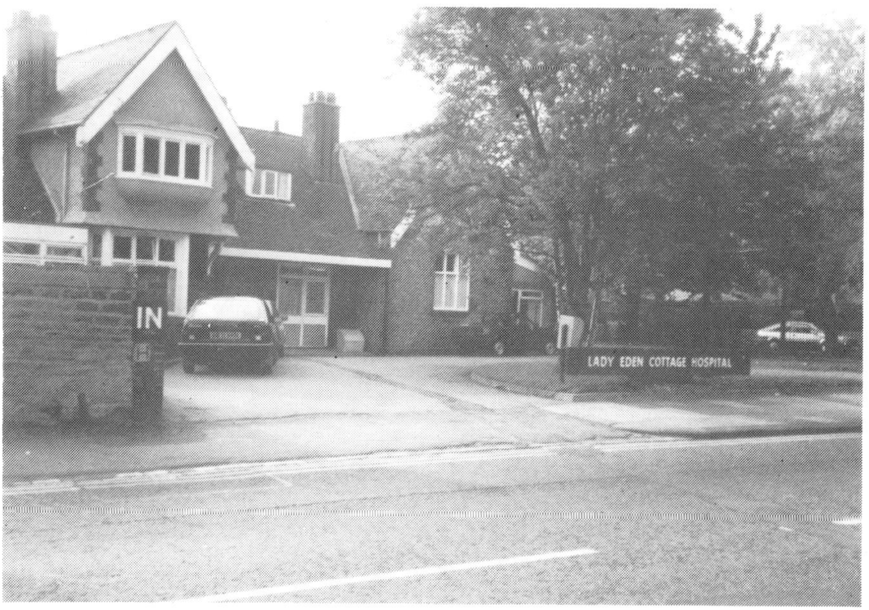

The Lady Eden Cottage Hospital in 1989.

The Children in the care of the Guardians in the Early Years of the 20th Century

Children were admitted if the family became destitute and the parents had to be admitted. Others were admitted with their mother who had been abandoned by the husband. Children were also admitted because they were neglected or had themselves been abandoned by their parents. In other cases the mother was admitted for delivery (often an unmarried girl) and the baby was born in the institution and sometimes remained there a considerable time.

Apart from the heating of the infants' ward and the organisation of one outing a year, little mention is made of the children until about 1900. The Rev Dean Little was now on the Board and he frequently asked questions about the children. The town committee arranged an outing for the children of the town and invited the workhouse children to join in the treat. They went in brakes to Witton Castle and the Guardians committee had a collection from those at the meeting and contributed 14/- towards the expenses.

Mrs J.T. Proud was a leading member of the ladies' committee and took a keen interest in the children. From time to time a woman would ask the Guardians to provide a girl to become her maidservant, or a farmer for a boy to be a farmhand. At other times a couple would ask if they could adopt a child. Mrs Proud began to assess these applications — they were normally dealt with by the Relieving Officer. She told the committee that she had seen the people concerned and inspected the premises, and that in some cases she approved and in others she did not approve, and the committee seemed to take her advice. Later when the cottage homes were opened, she took a close interest in the welfare of the children there.

From 1896 until 1930 the committee was involved in arrangements "to emigrate children to America". This was a national scheme supported by the churches of the day. The idea was to give the children a new home usually in Canada with a prospect of education, training and work. The children could refuse to go and had to be passed as medically fit. The Guardians paid the expenses and were responsible for the child until he or she became 18 years old. In 1911 the cost to send a boy of $15^1/_2$ years to Canada via the waifs and strays Church of England Society was £13 made up of: £4 for an outfit, 10/- railway fare to the port of embarkation (usually Liverpool), passage money, kit and bedding £4.10.0 and the remainder £4.0.0. as other expenses. The committee in 1896 agreed to send 10 boys — either orphans or deserted children to America. The arrangements were made through the Manchester and Salford aid society and also the Liverpool Catholic childrens protection society. From time to time other children were sent. On one occasion a boy of seven told the committee that he didn't want to go as he wished to become a farmer. He could not therefore be sent.

By 1901 the minutes were a little more graceful. It became the practice to send expressions of thanks to various people who gave help to inmates, children and patients. 26 children and 4 adult escorts were sent to Redcar. A piano was bought for £23. The floor of the lying in ward was covered in linoleum at the request of the visiting committee. Dr Wardle did not seem to be sending so many letters to the committee. Land on the north side of the institution was to be used as a cricket playing area for the boys.

Also in 1902 the local government board asked the Guardians what progress had been made to remove the children from the institution as suggested in 1898. No progress had in fact been made, but now the Guardians bought the land for £50 and in 1903 sent rough plans to the local government board for approval. Meanwhile an attempt to get all the children boarded out in separate houses was made. Three sisters aged 12, 10 and 8 were in fact boarded with families but each girl went to a different family and were to be regarded as "adopted" children.

Four cottage homes for the children were erected, the cost £6,000. Furniture was purchased and three foster mothers aged 25-30 years were appointed at a salary of £25 per year and one superintendent foster mother at £30 per year. The field around the homes was to be used as a playground and Dr Wardle would be paid £10 a year to look after the children (and provide all necessary drugs and dressings).

The four cottages are still there in Escomb Road on the hospital site opposite the new boiler house. They were opened in 1905. Each house had a foster mother in charge. Soon after they were opened Dr Wardle complained that there was no provision for a sick bay in one house to provide care for the children of all the houses in which to look after common mild childhood ailments.

Mrs Proud wrote him a letter. It was she said, the purpose in appointing a foster mother in each house to ensure that the children in each house, would remain under the care of one woman, as in a normal household. It followed that if a child fell ill and was not bad enough to be removed to hospital, he or she would remain under the care of his or her own foster mother, as in a normal house. Dr Wardle, she continued, must cease putting all the sick children together in one of the houses and must give to each foster mother instructions about the care of the child, and give into her hands, the necessary drugs and dressings, as he would do in any normal home in the district. Dr Wardle immediately agreed.

Mrs Proud also issued instructions about training the children. They attended local schools during the day although initially three girls had been refused admission to St. Anne's, the British school, and also the Wesleyan school, as there were no places then available.

An industrial trained and relief foster mother was appointed in 1912 to assist the foster mothers. She was to rise at 6 a.m. from March to September and at 6.45 a.m. during the remaining months. She slept in No. 1 house and had to divide her time equally between the four houses. She was to assist the

The people were transferred, but I do not know the final charge agreed.

About this time Dr Campbell, a member of the Board of Guardians objected to the use of the word "pauper" in connection with the inmates and it was agreed to try to avoid the use of the term.

Dr Wardle, in 1915, was appointed Lieutenant Colonel to the 6th Durhams stationed at Roker, Sunderland. He wrote to the committee saying that he would, however, continue to come regularly to do his work at the institution and that his deputy would help. The Board agreed.

Gradually more staff joined the services. In particular, the Superintendant Nurse — Miss Jackson joined up and was posted to Cairo. The committee thought highly of her and kept her post open although she offered to resign so that a permanent appointment could be made. When the war ended she wrote from Cairo that she intended to stay in the Army and though the committee tried to get her to change her mind they had to accept her decision.

By February, 1918, a further 50 soldiers beds were requested by the War Office. The committee agreed, but asked the War Office for help in providing nurses. Colonel Wardle said he was perfectly willing to look after any number of soldiers who were admitted. There are no details of the type of illness affecting the soldiers, but I think they were all from surrounding units in the area and mainly sick rather than suffering from war injuries, but this is uncertain. Acute surgical treatment was certainly concentrated in Newcastle.

On 14th November, 1918, three days after Armistice, the Guardians met and, on the motion of the chairman, the meeting started with the committee singing the Doxology and the National Anthem "as prayer and praise in respect of the signing of the Armistice on 11th November, 1918".

In these days and another war later this may seem unusual but not so I suspect, when I recollect how often the previous meetings had begun by referring to the death or injury of a former employee, inmate, or relative of a committee member.

By December, 1918, the military beds were closed. 1,154 patients had been treated in the previous two years and two months. Colonel Adams, AMS, i/c Northumberland war hospital thanked the Guardians. The hospital, he wrote, was always a favourite with his men, who often asked to be admitted to Bishop Auckland institution rather than elsewhere and the men had been looked after splendidly.

1918 Onwards to the 1939 War

After the war financial troubles began. In 1921 the bank refused to honour a cheque for £1,000 presented by a relieving officer to allow him to provide statutory help. The directors of the bank required the permission of the Ministry of Health to allow them to grant an extension of the overdraft. The clerk to the Guardians issued a cheque for £1,000 from his private account to enable the relieving officer to assist a number of people and telegraphed the Ministry of Health for a £10,000 increase in overdraft until a full statement of affairs could be presented, but by January, 1922, a further £25,000 was needed and granted.

In the same year the Guardians were asked to pay travelling expenses for the girls boarded at St. Mary's Home, Tudhoe, to visit their brothers who were at St. Peter's Home, Gainford. This was refused. Patients receiving electrical treatment as out-patients were asked to pay five shillings per attendance. Dr Wardle wanted an x-ray unit installed costing £490. This was refused. However, the Bishop Auckland Cottage Hospital offered the use of their x-ray. It would cost ten shillings without a plate (i.e. film) and fifteen shillings with a plate together with five shillings for a further examination without a plate. This was accepted.

The committee reviewed the hours of work of the nurses in 1923. The night charge nurse worked from 8.30 p.m. to 7.30 a.m. six nights a week. The day charge nurse worked from 8.00 a.m. with 2 hours off, a four day week, there was one whole day of 11 hours off, one evening of $2^1/_2$ hours and on Sundays they had off duty periods of $3^1/_2$ and 6 hours on alternative weeks. The probationers started at 7.00 a.m. and worked until 8.30 p.m. with 2 hours off on five days a week and one whole day off. On Sundays $3^1/_2$ hours off was allowed in the morning on Sunday and $3^1/_2$ hours in the evening on the next Sunday.

The committee, having considered these hours decided they should be continued. They changed the title charge nurse to that of sister. They also decided to start a nurses training school but this proved to be difficult as the General Nursing Council thought the experience the nurses gained was too limited. Eventually in 1925 a linkage was established with Wingrove Hospital, later the Newcastle General Hospital. The nurses started training at Bishop Auckland and after two years went to the Wingrove for a further two years. This arrangement lasted until 1933 when the Wingrove withdrew from the scheme.

By 1925 the Ministry said that they did not approve the employment of girls under the age of nineteen years as probationer nurses, and that although those now in post at eighteen years could continue, new applicants must be nineteen years or over.

The care of patients suffering from tuberculosis had become a local authority duty in 1913, but by 1925 the newly appointed tuberculosis Medical Officer for the county refused to transfer patients with tuberculosis in the institution to sanatoria or elsewhere. The committee decided to erect some wooden chalets, they were not to have an interior lining and no heating was to be provided. Each chalet held two patients. These huts were modelled on those used at Holywood Hall. The Ministry of Health at first refused to sanction them, saying that the outdoor treatment was only of value in early cases, but quite useless in advanced cases. Dr Wardle disagreed and finally the Ministry said, that though they still could not agree the principle, they would not oppose the erection of the huts.

Dr Mark Wardle died suddenly on the 14th April, 1926, and was succeeded by his son Dr V.H. Wardle. Dr Val as he was known, reported in 1928 that he was now treating a poor law patient with insulin because of diabetes. He was requested by the committee to report on the condition of the patient in three months time and meanwhile as he had supplied the insulin he was to receive 10/6d per week to cover the cost and later the Ministry approved the payment.

New Ideas but Little Progress

After the Board of Guardians were abolished in 1930, all the poor law institutions came under the control of the Durham County Council Public Assistance Committee and the Auckland institution was in No. 1 (Auckland) area. The new committee surveyed all the institutions. There were in the Auckland institution in 1930, 326 beds made up by 99 for able bodied adults (23 vacant) 119 for sick inmates (48 vacant) maternity beds 4 — all vacant, 83 mental deficiency patients were housed from Prudhoe mental colony (one vacant) and there were 21 children's beds (18 vacant). In addition 62 beds were available in the cottage homes, but only 27 were occupied and one home was closed. Thus 259 beds were occupied and 129 vacant.

The County Council Committee decided that all the poor law buildings were obsolete and incapable of being adapted to present day requirements. They purchased two sites — Dryburn estate (48 acres) for £16,500 and West Lodge estate (14½ acres) for £5,500. They intended to build a new central hospital on these sites in Durham to provide one hospital for the whole county. Discussions were held with representatives of the voluntary hospitals in Newcastle, Sunderland, Darlington, Durham and Stockton and the building of the new hospital was supported provided that there was no interference with the work of the voluntary hospitals. This was in 1930.

Thereafter, despite much discussion and repeated resolutions stressing the great need for better facilities nothing much happened.

It was agreed that the new Dryburn site hospital would take time to materialise and in 1932 alternative schemes were considered. There were some 808 beds available in the county of which about 650 were usually occupied and in addition the cottage homes of the county, provided another 692 beds of which 150 were usually vacant. Dr A.E. Raine had joined the staff of the Medical Officer of Health in 1930 and he now suggested that the only council health building in all the council, institutions, that could be regarded as reasonably suitable for modern medical and surgical treatment was the Bishop Auckland Infirmary. (Previously all the buildings were regarded as obsolete). But, he said, the beds would be limited to 118 for surgical cases, a lift would be needed together with considerable alterations. A nurses' home would be required (up to now nurses often had rooms adjoining each ward). He also thought that Chester-le-Street institution should be closed. The cottage homes would become nurses homes. It was said that Bishop Auckland had a good operating theatre and that if the mentally defective patients who came from other areas were relocated the 118 beds could increase to 160. These would be used for surgical patients plus an out-patient department and an electrical department. The unit was separated from the institution and could have a special entrance from either Escomb Road or Westfield Road. Maternity cases would go to Durham Public Assistance Hospital. The management would be by a special committee and then the patients would not need to seek admission through the poor law system and hence avoid the stigma. The Ministry approved these suggestions and did not feel that a new hospital at Dryburn needed all 500 beds. The need for orthopaedic beds for the treatment of surgical tuberculosis was stressed. The cost would be about £29,200. Nothing much happened.

In 1934 the Ministry reviewed the Dryburn plan and suggested members of the committee should visit other counties where similar hospitals had been built. The visits were made, the planned number of beds at Dryburn were reduced from 500 to 300 in the first instance and in 1935 the Ministry approved this idea, but now hoped that the needs for materinity beds would be considered. The voluntary hospitals became alarmed. They asked how the patients would be admitted, how would the units be staffed and what would be the effect on voluntary hospitals? They, the voluntary hospitals, wanted only poor law patients to be admitted to the new Dryburn hospital.

No progress over the Dryburn site hospital or the various suggestions of surgical beds at Bishop Auckland and medical beds at Chester-le-Street was made. Whenever redecoration or rebuilding was suggested at Bishop Auckland the idea was usually shelved in view of the forthcoming changes.

Meanwhile, by 1936 more male beds were needed at Bishop Auckland. There were 47 male patients but only 37 beds. The era of overcrowding was beginning. The nurses slept in side rooms and on the male wards and it was thought that if they could be moved to a nurses home an additional 5 beds could be provided for male patients.

However, eventually, some redecoration, with extensions to the kitchen were carried out and two childrens homes were taken over for nurses accommodation. The total cost of this was £2,503.

In 1938 eight years after it was first suggested, the cost of the Dryburn project was estimated at £345,000. The Commissioner for Special Areas was asked to provide 85% of this and in June, 1938, he agreed, but stressed that the grant would only be paid if work was started at once, otherwise the money would be used elsewhere. This produced activity. No quantity surveyors could be found in the north east who could do the work in time to

Health and administered by the Regional Health Authority. Oaklands institution was then used mainly for hospital purposes and hence was transferred from the County Council to the Regional Health Authority and became a hospital. There were, however, 23 non sick public assistance people still left in the hospital. These were always referred to as Part 3 inmates.

The first meeting of the South West Durham Hospital Management Committee was held in June, 1948, at the council offices, Glenholme, Crook. Alderman F. Hunt was Chairman. It was agreed to advertise the post of Secretary/Finance Officer to the Management Committee and thereafter the other necessary officers. Oaklands Hospital would in future be called the Bishop Auckland General Hospital.

Mr K.G.T. Luxford started as HMC Secretary/Finance Officer on 20th September, 1948. The EMS huts were largely empty as the German P.O.Ws. had returned home. The equipment was badly worn. It was thought that 200-300 new beds would have to be bought to replace the narrow collapsible emergency beds and this would cost about £70,000. The General Hospital was inspected and a list of urgent works required was made. Some parts were dangerous, others suffered from flooding. The laundry chimney which served no useful purpose was dangerous and needed removal. There were many other serious matters. The County Architect agreed to deal with the most urgent work. Dr A.E. Raine was already in post as Medical Superintendent. He was transferred to the NHS and in September, 1948, he also was appointed Assistant Senior Administrative Medical Officer to the Regional Hospital Board, a post which took up one third of his time. Miss Dinning the Superintendent Nurse at the institution, was taken over as Matron at the General Hospital. Hospital maintenance left much to be desired and a Handyman/Joiner and a Handyman/Mason were appointed. In December, 1948, Mr T. Robinson was appointed Hospital Engineer. There were mentally defective women housed in the hospital and the Regional Health Authority was asked to consider transferring them to Binchester Whins Hospital which was empty.

Apart from a small amount of general surgery, there was little acute work done in the hospital and gradually the beds became filled with long stay nursing problems. The only casualty service in 1948 was provided at the Lady Eden Hospital by a rota of general practitioners. As the beds at the Lady Eden were not fully used, it was agreed that part of the hospital should be used for ENT cases — mainly removal of tonsils and adenoids, by Mr J.S. Monro. Dr H.A. Dewar had an appointment as consultant physician to Durham County Council poor law institution and used to visit Bishop Auckland one day a month.

It was already clear that there were too many infectious disease beds in the district and hence it was agreed that Helmington Row Hospital would gradually be altered to receive geriatric patients from the General Hospital and then allow Blocks 2 and 3 to be rebuilt. 14 beds would, however, be retained for the case of advanced pulmonary tuberculosis. Weardale Isolation Hospital at Stanhope was rarely used and it was suggested that it should be used as a sanatorium for tuberculosis. This did not occur and the hospital was finally closed in 1952. It had been virtually empty for 2-3 years previously.

Plans for a new hospital in Bishop Auckland were made. In 1948 the Regional Health Board thought the hospital should be demolished and replaced by a new 500 bedded hospital on the same site. As this would be a costly long term plan, Messrs. Millburn the Sunderland Architects drew up an interim plan for a 200 bedded hospital. It centred on seven hutted wards together with Blocks 1 and 2. Out-patient facilities and a nurse training school and other special departments including 20 beds for midwifery in Block 1 were to be provided, together with the conversion of one hutted ward to a childrens' ward. Much of this plan ultimately was provided, but the original 500 bed plan never got under way.

When I was appointed in 1949, I was shown a delightful plan and model of the new hospital and told that all the existing buildings would be replaced. Though many alterations and some new buildings have been erected, the old blocks and huts still remain some 40 years later.

Attempts were made to get the County Council to remove the non sick public assistance cases in the so called part 3 accommodation, but without success. Indeed the County Council asked for more men to be admitted but this was refused.

In mid 1949 the newly formed Medical Advisory Committee, composed mainly of general practitioners, and specialists in tuberculosis together with the surgeons and anaesthetists from Darlington discussed visiting to the children in hospitals. The committee advised the HMC that routine visiting of children was not desirable because:

1. there was risk of introducing infection
2. parents gave children unsuitable things to eat
3. children became very upset when parents leave.

However, it was agreed that seriously ill children should be visited and that children in hospitals for infectious diseases (the "fever hospitals") could have a visitor for ten minutes on a Saturday, but not until the child had been in hospital a few days and had time to settle down.

I was appointed in 1949 but could not be released by the RVI until 1st February, 1950, but at the request of Dr Dewar was able to replace him and came down to see out-patients once a week for a few months before February, 1950.

The hutted wards H and J were designated for medical use but they were full of long stay surgical cases and it took some months before they were available for acute medical admissions. Even then 6 male and 3 female beds were used for orthopaedic patients. Neither ward, nor the childrens ward, had much in the way of basic equipment or drugs to deal with acute emergencies. Together with the ward sisters a new inventory was drawn up and gradually the necessary items were obtained. These included blood pressure machines, thermometers and the necessary medical equipment for examination and treatment of the patients.

The stigma of the workhouse, prevented many patients agreeing to come to the hospital for treatment and I was often told "you only go there to die". However, gradually this changed and patients discovered they could be investigated, treated and recover.

The nursing staff in the ward consisted of one sister, one staff nurse and the rest were assistant nurses. There was no training school for nurses. Nevertheless the basic nursing care was good and extremely kind. The pace of work was slow — much more so than I had been used to at the RVI. If I suggested to Sister that a patient should go home, she would often say "yes, I agree, but let me see, today is Thursday, well she (the patient) cannot go home until after the weekend as there's the shopping to do, the room to be prepared and the bed aired. Do you think we should arrange an ambulance for next Tuesday or Wednesday or would that be too soon?" It took some time to speed up the process. Meanwhile no one else could be admitted to that bed. Nevertheless it was very important to work with the staff and not against them as they were genuinely concerned with the welfare of their patients and grew to welcome the essential changes.

At the beginning of the NHS a great deal of ill health was revealed. This was also so in S.W. Durham. The hutted wards of the EMS Hospital together with Blocks 1 and 2 of the former institution held many patients with chronic diseases for which no cure existed. In addition there were many people in the community with similar diseases. Some of the latter were awaiting admission to hospital.

There was a waiting list for the long stay beds, which was handed to me when I arrived. In the book were written some notes concerning patients wishing to be admitted. Sometimes there was a name, age, address, diagnosis and the name of the general practitioner. These are the normal requirements. However, such detail was rarely present. Sometimes there was only a name, at times a name and address. Occasionally the note merely said Councillor "X's" man or Rev. "Y's" man. From time to time a doctors name was added. It was impossible to organise a proper admission system with this inadequate information and I decided that in future admissions would only be considered at the request of a general practitioner. As I met doctors I showed them the list I had, and an odd patient was identified. Frequently he or she had been dealt with or was dead. Usually I was then given the names and details of another person who needed admission.

As beds became available — mainly by discharge of surgical patients inhabiting the two wards H and J that were designated for medical patients. I was able to start dealing with the waiting list. The number of people requiring admission rapidly rose — chiefly elderly people. In addition to requests from general practitioners for admission, in the early months I also received demands from a few councillors who felt they had lost "their" hospital and the authority to try to admit patients. At times businessmen demanded admission of a relative or their personal secretary or someone similar who was off work caring for an aged relative. This was not to benefit the patient, who often did not wish to be admitted, but to enable the executive to carry out his work. Occasionally hints of bribery were made to expedite admission. On other occasions threats were issued. One important local dignitary threatened to report me to his friend Mr Aneurin Bevan. I said that I hoped the man would do so and ask Mr Bevan to provide more money for the hospitals and also to visit it and especially Block 3. There was no reply and no action.

This shortage of chronic beds for elderly people was a national problem and the newspapers constantly reported the failure of hospitals to admit such patients. Yet if the beds were full and the nursing staff too few there really was nothing one could do except to press on with changes and obtain more and better accommodation. Putting up extra beds in already overcrowded wards was not a real solution.

Slowly we got more beds, the Management Committee and all the hospital staff were anxious and determined to improve the situation. Helmington Row Hospital stopped admitting infectious diseases and was gradually altered to admit elderly chronic sick. It was more difficult to get Tindale Crescent Hospital closed for infectious diseases. Doctors and local councillors said that infectious disease beds were essential. I was eventually able to show that only two practices sent patients into the hospital. One of the practices concerned only sent children in from a residential establishment. When the authorities of this charity were approached, they gladly agreed to provide a sick bay to look after the children with rubella, chicken pox or scarlet fever, if I would agree to deal with any more serious cases. The remaining practice was one of two in a small town. The other practice in the town never found it necessary to send children with more common infections to hospital but the social conditions of the patients in the two practices were exactly the same. When these facts were explained the medical opposition to closure of Tindale Crescent disappeared and we were able to start to alter the wards.

Other things of course were happening. The buildings of the General Hospital — as it was now called, were old and in need of restoration and repair. The hutted wards also needed improvements. There were no side wards. Heating of the huts was still by means of coke stoves refilled 3 or 4 times in 24 hours as mentioned previously.

In June, 1950, the hospital laundry was declared to be too dangerous for use. The factory inspectorate agreed. The laundry was closed and a private firm awarded the contract. This privatisation did not arouse any opposition and continued until a new laundry was built at Aycliffe Hospital and opened in the late 1960's.

Blocks 2 and 3 in the 1950's

Block 2 was rather depressing. Downstairs there was a ward with elderly women, some demented, others paralysed. In one room there were three mentally defective patients, now adults but referred to as children, who had been born in the Institution. They had spina bifide and hydrocephalus. They had been abandoned by their relatives and were totally unable to do anything for themselves.

The ward itself was painted and seemed to be a brownish grey. The artificial light was inadequate. There was virtually no possibility of discharging any of the patients, and visitors were a great rarity and most patients had not been visited for some years. This state of affairs continued until I reported to the Hospital Management Committee that one night rats ran over the beds. The ward was shut and the patients moved upstairs to a lighter ward.

Gloomy though Block 2 was, it was bright and cheerful when compared to Block 3. This large block, housed downstairs about 23 part 3 inmates — the ambulant non sick waiting to transfer to County Council residential accommodation. It had also been the Tramp Reception Centre. Upstairs was the chronic sick male ward containing about 80 patients. The rooms were not connected by a corridor but each room led onto the next. The painting on the walls where it existed, was dirty brown. The floor was uneven and wooden. Some parts had a linoleum cover. The steps up to the second floor were stone and severely worn and hollowed, but also sloped downwards so that they were very unsafe. Rickety iron gates were in place at the top and bottom of each staircase but rarely closed properly. The toilets were totally inadequate in number, rarely had any seats and were chipped and cracked. There were only two or three baths and about six wash handbasins. The sluice rooms were dark small and primitive and the small kitchen had worn out equipment. The steep staircase had a narrow turn at the top. Nurses have told me that because of this the corpses had to be held upright to enable them to be carried down the stairs to proceed to the mortuary.

All the beds were crowded together so that if a patient in the centre of the ward needed attention many beds had to be moved so the nurse or myself had to sidle between beds to reach the desired one. There were no chairs or lockers between the beds — there was no room. No screens were provided and they could not have been used had there been any as there was no room. Only thin nurses could work on the ward. The lighting was not adequate. One single electric light bulb hung nakedly in the centre of each ward and one — about 60 watts sufficed in one ward for about 20 beds. The windows fitted badly, rattled and let in wind and rain. At the extreme south end was one room sardonically called a ward. It held six beds. The plaster had fallen off the southern wall and several square feet of bricks were exposed. The plaster between the bricks had disappeared in places and clouds, sky and rain could be seen. The normal complement for such a sized room would be two beds, possibly three in an emergency. The roof leaked and dishes had to be put in position and one bed covered with a mackintosh.

Overall this there was the smell. This was a complex odour but fragments could be recognised. It was made up of human excrement, the odour of bodies, decaying damp plaster, rotting wood, cockroaches, beetles, mice, cats and possibly rats. It was a distinctive powerful and disgusting stench.

There were no flowers, decorations, pictures or photographs. There was indeed nowhere to put them and no one would have attempted to hang a picture as more plaster would have fallen off.

No visitors ever came, the patients were admitted and abandoned. Senior staff came in rarely. I tried to go round three and four times a week but it took a long time before I could say that I had properly examined all the patients. There were virtually no hospital notes in the accepted sense.

To nurse these patients there were three or four disabled male nurses and occasionally female nurses helped. Overall was the Sister-in-Charge — a small slight woman. She was a remarkable person. She came on duty each day in these appalling conditions and fought to improve the lot of her patients and seemed always, when I arrived, to be doing battle with some-one in Authority — frequently the person responsible for sending the single weekly treat of 1-2 ozs. tobacco for the patients. This was their only plea-sure, and without Sisters remorseless prompting they would have been deprived even of that. She struggled to give what nursing care was possible. Despite all this she remained cheerful and did not seem to wish to move to another ward. Eventually in 1952 she did resign to look after her aging mother.

The first task was to empty the six bedded end ward. Eventually a patient died and this bed was removed. This left more space for the buckets and dishes. Gradually the patients died or I was able to move them elsewhere and that ward was shut and the door locked. As I examined the other patients one or two seemed likely to benefit from treatment. Four men had had supra-pubic bladder drainage because of prostate enlargement but the second stage operation — to remove the prostate had been deemed impos-sible.

Mr John Swinney then the Consultant Urological Surgeon in Newcastle kindly agreed to help and though the only had six beds he slowly took each of these patients, removed, in one case with considerable difficulty, the prostate and they came back to recuperate and all four eventually were dis-charged home or to hostels. A new treatment for Parkinsons disease was appearing — Artane — and Professor Nattrass, my old chief, asked if I would like to try it and let him know the result. It was not yet available generally. I tried it on three or four patients and gradually built the dose up — we didn't know how best to use it. The result was startling. One man began to walk round the Hospital grounds for the first time in a year or two. The dose used was some twenty times the dose now recommended. The other cases were dramatically improved but none was cured. Unfortunately the toxic side effects then appeared, fever and confusion especially, and the dose had to be reduced and the patients relapsed. Nevertheless these trials had important effect in improving the morale of the patients in the ward and the staff.

It was clear, however, that the whole building would need closing and we hoped that Helmington Row Hospital would take most of the patients — but not those categorised in part 3 — the ambulant poor law patients.

In February 1962 Mr Robinson, the Hospital Engineer and I walked past the building in the evening after a meeting of a sub-committee of the HMC. We agreed that the roof appeared to be sagging and Mr Robinson inspected this the next day and reported that the building was dangerous and must be closed. This was decisive. The County Council found space for their men, Helmington Row took most of the patients and ward 7 — a hutted ward took the remainder. This squalid building was at last empty.

Shortly afterwards the roof was removed for replacement. Promptly on the following Saturday night the north and gable wall collapsed.

I have written perhaps a little bitterly about the ward but I do not think I exaggerate. Dr Patterson the Senior Administration Medical Officer of the Regional Board told me that he thought it was the worst block in the region. Dr (later Sir) James Spence the distinguished Physician and Professor of Child Health at Newcastle used to bring visiting Doctors from various parts of the world to see it and mischievously encouraged them to take a deep breath as they entered.

How did such a situation develop?

I think there were several reasons, all cumulative.

One was shortage of money — especially between the two World Wars in the era of depression and great unemployment, (up to 40% in this area). Another was the feeling that the poor law patients were partly to blame for their situation — though this was lessening in the 1930's. Yet another was the inertia over the two plans for the county poor law patients — either to push on with the Dryburn plan or to go for the split site — Chester-le-Street and Bishop Auckland plan as already mentioned. This led to the failure to spend enough money on the maintenance of the existing buildings and it deflected interest in the slowly developing decay. Then of course the 1939-45 war prevented all but essential war work and after the war, the shortage and the 1946 embargo on Hospital building, in order to concentrate on building houses, accelerated the decay. In addition, the County Council was, I imagine, reluctant to spend money on a building that was to be taken off them at the start of the NHS.

Over and above all these important reasons was another — psychological. The public as a whole took little interest in poor law activities, the visiting committee rarely went round the whole Hospital and I suspect they often saw only parts that they were shown by the Master and Matron or their staff. The Committee had no experience of the Hospitals and technical, engineering and medical advice was in short supply. Advances in medicine and surgery were taking place in the Teaching Hospitals, but their medical and nursing staffs rarely, if ever, saw the poor law staff or establishments. The slow decay of the fabric went unnoticed. The enclosed life in the institution was not exposed to the public gaze.

Brian Abel-Smith in his account of the first thirty years of the National Health Service quoted a distinguished doctor saying that the Poor Law Hospitals at the start of the NHS, apart from a few notable exceptions, remained "ill designed, deficient in sanitation, often isolated, bare, bleak and soulless".

The Hutted Wards

In July, 1950, I was able to start a series of clinical meetings with general practitioners. These took place on Sunday mornings and general practitioners came from a wide area to see certain patients in the wards and discuss the diagnosis and treatment. Although I was nominally the teacher, I always thought that I learned much more from these meetings than the general practitioners did. It was fascinating to hear the discussions that arose. Many doctors present would know various relations of the actual patient and a pattern of diseases in the families would emerge which was not mentioned in the textbooks. No one received any payment for these courses and several doctors travelled long distances to attend. The patients and staff were very cooperative and we all felt this was not only a method of learning but incidentally improved the morale of the hospital. I look back on those early days of learning with particular pleasure.

Indeed, despite the poor physical surroundings, the shortages, the lack of equipment, the low staff/patient ratio and the almost complete absence of any of the usual ancillary services, it was an exciting time. The newly appointed Consultants were young and enthusiastic and like all grades of staff were determined to make the new NHS work. Everyone felt a new era was beginning.

There was indeed, a great deal to do. Although nowadays the hospitals are praised rightly, for the vast increase in "through put" or turn over of patients, this has been done with vastly improved hospital premises, many more staff and much more elaborate technological help.

I am not of course denigrating these improvements which indeed are remarkable. But it is I think equally remarkable to consider how a very small staff, with very inadequate resources and little technological help could transform a static hospital into a busy acute unit and still provide long term care. These developments were not unique to Bishop Auckland, they took place in all the hospitals.

Dr W. Walker was appointed as first full-time Radiologist to the hospital in 1950. The Maternity Unit was planned to be in the upper floor of Block 1 and an Out-Patient and Casualty Department in the ground floor, south end. These were ready in 1951. Prior to that Mr D. Galloway was appointed in mid February, 1950, to assist Mr Hovell, Consultant Obstetrician and Gynaecologist. When Block 1 Maternity Unit was open, it was intended that Mr Hovell would work entirely at Darlington and Northallerton and this took place and Mr Galloway took charge at Bishop Auckland. Meanwhile, temporary changes were made in ward K — which was intended to be the childrens ward, to provide Maternity Unit accommodation. The County Maternity Home in Princes Street was of course functioning under Mr Galloway with the local general practitioner sharing three beds.

Plans to improve all the hospitals in the Group were made and as money became available they were gradually executed, but little or nothing was heard of the master plan to rebuild the whole hospital in Bishop Auckland.

By June, 1951, the government was in financial difficulties and the first of the now familiar financial cuts occurred.

In the meeting that month the Management Committee had to defer the upgrading of Block 3, the opening of a new ante natal ward, the opening of Block 4 as a nurses home, the re-opening after alterations of a 20 bedded ward at Holywood Hall Hospital and the admission of 15 geriatric patients to Homelands Hospital (formerly Helmington Row Hospital).

Gradually these restrictions were lifted and further improvements planned. The hospital kitchen which was old and had poor equipment was shut and the kitchen in the hutted complex used in its place.

There was great difficulty in getting staff of all grades and this was partly due to lack of housing. The Management Committee therefore began to rent houses in the new Dene Hall Estate as they were built. Later the committee bought houses near to the hospital — chiefly in Westfield Road and converted them into small flats. At one time it was said that we had more married accommodation for junior hospital doctors than any other hospital in North East England and this certainly helped in recruitment. Prior to the NHS, junior hospital doctors were rarely married and hence lived in the hospital.

Bishop Auckland was allocated one of three civil defence wards in the Region. The new building became Ward 4 — orthopaedic — and in March, 1952, Mr A.B. McCulloch was appointed Consultant Orthopaedic

Surgeon. Mr E.P. Waters who had been doing the work in addition to orthopaedic duties in Darlington now gave up Bishop Auckland and returned to Darlington. It soon became clear that more operating theatres were needed, together with more anaesthetic staff and more nurses. The easiest part was the building, though it seemed a long wait for its creation. However, it was opened by Mr Gordon Irwin head of the orthopaedic department at the R.V.I. in 1958. The shortage of staff continued long after that.

An important development occurred in 1952. Professor Nattrass, Professor of Medicine at Newcastle, called a group of Physicians working in the region or "peripheral" hospitals to a meeting one Friday afternoon. I think there were about eight of us. We were invited to accept two medical students for a months residence in our hospitals during January, February and March of each year. We were asked to arrange residence for them in the hospital and give them access to the patients under our care and to teach them. The idea was that they would get more intensive personal tuition and see acute diseases at any time of day or night. The HMC and administrative staff welcomed the suggestion. The students lived in the top storey of the Lady Eden Hospital and seemed to enjoy and appreciate the experience they gained. This was probably the first formal attachment of students from the University to such hospitals in the country. It was quickly followed elsewhere except in London where it was only slowly accepted. We had a constant supply of students and usually a waiting list for other students to come. Later obstetrical, paediatric and surgical students came under the same scheme.

Again the stimulation of teaching students raised standards of medical care. Several former students still tell me of their enjoyable time spent at Bishop Auckland.

Gordon Cameron came as Consultant Surgeon in 1953 and for the first time we had an active young surgeon resident in the town. He was making great progress and transformed the surgical side of the hospital before his untimely, sudden death on 19th July, 1955.

Slowly but surely more improvements to the buildings occurred. Central heating was installed and as this called for the ward to be shut, the opportunity was taken to improve the ward at the same time. Thus there was always, for many years, one ward out of use for upgrading purposes. The need for side wards was recognised and here voluntary organisations helped greatly. Amongst others, the Shildon Railways Employees Hospital and Motor Ambulance Association gave £1,000 to the hospital to provide side wards. A League of Hospital Friends was established in 1952 and gradually gave invaluable help. Sections of the League were formed at Homelands and Tindale Crescent Hospitals and have provided a great deal of help in those hospitals. In addition many other people and numerous organisations have helped from time to time. When we started in 1948 there were no endowment funds at the General Hospital, now there are quite valuable funds available. These provide special items of equipment and give extra comfort and help to the patient. There is no sign of lessening of this kindly and generous spirit.

The ancillary services needed to increase and the first resident Consultant Pathologist was appointed to replace Dr Hurwicz who came over from Sedgefield. Dr J.M. Robertson started in May, 1952, and began to develop the modern Pathology Unit.

There were national shortages of trained staff and of course this was reflected locally. Consultants in several specialities — anaesthetics, paediatrics, geriatrics, radiology and casualty were all in very short supply. There were similar shortages of physiotheraptists, occupational therapists, dieticians, laboratory technicians and social workers and even when money was available, they could not be recruited.

Miss L. Dyke had arrived to help Mr. Galloway and for a few years worked at Dryburn and Bishop Auckland. Mr H.M. Jamison had become Senior Casualty Officer and in October, 1955, was appointed with Mr Wrigley as Consultant General Surgeon. The pair of them worked tirelessly to produce a remarkable surgical unit and provide the type of service the NHS was always intended to produce — effective care by Consultants themselves, of all the patients.

The childrens ward was of course a mixed ward of medical and surgical cases. The visiting hours had been set by the HMC on the advice of the then Medical Advisory Committee as already mentioned. The Ministry of Health recommended in 1953 that all children should be visited by their parents. I had been pressing for a year or two for better visiting hours. The other Consultants were doubtful about increased visiting and the nursing staff were generally opposed, as were most nurses in the country.

The matter was discussed at a meeting of the Hospital Management Committee. Most of the lay members and especially the lady members were opposed to the extension of visiting. I finally had to say that if more visiting was not permitted I would record on the prescription sheet the instruction that the child under my care could have daily visiting, despite the fact that other children might not be visited. The meeting was perfectly friendly and the members of the committee were quite genuine in the belief that they were acting in the best interest of the children. However, they agreed to extend the visiting hours to each afternoon of the week, but at Tindale Crescent, which was still an infectious diseases hospital, visiting was restricted to $1^1/_2$ hours two afternoons a week. Nowadays of course the climate has changed and parents are welcome at almost any time in the childrens ward and some are able to stay overnight if they wish. Many hospitals in the country still have restrictions on visiting children. However, it is a slow job to change medical and surgical practice.

From 1955 onwards nursing staff shortages became more apparent.

Looking back over the Minutes of all the hospitals in the Group there has never been a time when there was not a nursing shortage, in the early years this was because the Guardians refused to employ more but after that it was because suitable applicants with the right training could not be recruited. The fact that during training a great many — sometimes up to 30% left for various reasons before completing the training, and others left soon after they qualified, made the position worse. In 1955 the Midwifery Department at the General Hospital and Princes Street Maternity Home were particularly affected.

The Family Planning Clinic began in 1957 in the Maternity Unit staffed by the Family Planning Association. There were strict criteria to be applied to the women seeking advice.

In October, 1957, the hospital like many others had to deal with the Asian Flu epidemic. All routine admissions were halted. The medical wards were completely taken over by Asian Flu victims and nurses were moved from the surgical and other departments to the medical wards and usually survived for a day or two before becoming patients themselves and going home. Volunteers came in from the town to assist with cooking and ward work and ex nurses returned to give whatever hours of work they could. Without this generous response from the community it is unlikely that the hospital could have managed. The main complication was staphyloccal pneumonia for which no antibiotic at that time was known. The disease could be extremely rapid in its progress. One lady went to serve in her shop at 9 a.m., was admitted to hospital by 11.30 a.m. and was dead by midday of bronchopneumonia. The epidemic subsided and life gradually got back to normal. The Hospital Management Committee issued a press statement thanking the public for all the help they had given. All the staff — but especially the nurses, had worked hard and the spirit was excellent.

In the same year 1957 Miss Dinning retired as Matron and a succession of Acting Matrons were then in post until Miss Vallack was appointed in May, 1958. Dr G. Ismay joined the Consultant Medical staff in the same month and like Miss Dyke worked at Dryburn Hospital and Bishop Auckland.

The Boardroom of the old institution is now the Assembly Hall. When in use as a Boardroom it was equipped with massive seating in semi circles around three wooden thrones for the Chairman and two Senior Officers. It had a double door at the entrance which led into a coloured glass canopy with side doors to prevent draughts and noise. It looked impressive. Each seat on the benches had a desk in front with an inkwell. All the seats and desks were of course firmly united to each other and access to the middle of the row already occupied by members was difficult. However, the acoustics were poor, the immovable furniture meant that movement was restricted and that the room despite its Victorian splendour could only be used for a few hours a week and sometimes less. Small committees were held in an adjoining room. In 1959 this furniture was removed, the ceiling lowered and the room has been used for many purposes since then. I have been unable to discover how much money was obtained for the sale of the furniture. Nowadays it would probably be of value.

The corridors of the hospital had all been open to the air up to 1959, but this posed dangers for unconscious patients leaving the hot operating theatres and gradually they were enclosed flooring material was fitted to cover the cement floor and the corridors were decorated. All this was completed by 1961.

Changes had eventually been made to Block 3. A new roof and gable end had been erected but then the building stood idle and empty, though gradually the ground floor was rebuilt. This was not without difficulty, because at one time the contractor said it was too dangerous — the building was likely to collapse. However, the Regional Health Authority provided more money so that steel girders could be inserted and work went ahead. The north end was converted into a small but useful geriatric day unit, the south end downstairs and upstairs were each converted into wards of 12 beds together with ancillary rooms, and a lift was installed. Mr Boyden the Member of Parliament for Bishop Auckland opened the Unit in September, 1961. The north end of the second floor was not developed but was closed off and used for storage purposes. Its condition was never as bad as the southern end.

Up to now the hospital had been the site of intensive building activity, replacing, improving and modifying existing buildings and occasionally adding small pieces. It was the only thing to do to make the hospital safe and to give a reasonable standard of service in all departments. Yet it was not satisfactory in some respects. There was a feeling that the more buildings were improved, the more likely it would be that they would be allowed to remain, and the real aim, mentioned in 1950, of a completely new modern hospital was being deferred and then still further deferred. There were a small number of voices heard opposing modification in order to heighten the claims for urgency in new buildings. However, when it was seen that nearly all the hospitals in North East England to say nothing of the rest of the country, were in the same plight it was obvious that rebuilding all the hospitals simultaneously was impossible. The main social priority was still the production of houses and factories. However, the programme of improvement continued and Mr Luxford the Group Secretary was very skilful in gathering round himself a small team who planned improvements to wards and departments in all the hospitals in the Group. These plans were often made even though no financial provision had been provided. However, it was quite common for money which had not been spent by the Regional Health Authority, to become available towards the end of the financial year provided it could be spent by 31st March. Because the plans were already made, Mr Luxford, almost every year was able to draw on this supply and get schemes carried through. The money came from the allocation of other Management Committees. In this way Bishop Auckland managed more quickly than many hospitals to level up the standards in all departments and got a reputation for doing so.

This unending work, however, imposed strain on the staff and patients. In thirty years I do not think that I was able to visit all the wards under my care in the various hospitals and not find one closed or partially out of action while workmen were changing them. However, each time a ward was upgraded some new idea was produced. It meant that as the demands of medical and surgical care also was rapidly changing they could at least in part be matched by building alterations. This is not possible in recently built multi-storey hospitals.

New Plans

In 1962 the Government produced a new hospital plan — the Blue Book. Ordinary hospital maintenance was some ten years in arrears, new hospitals were essential and the plan tried to look ten years ahead. The Blue Book seemed sensible and gave new hope to those wanting a new hospital. In the planning of new hospitals, however, one difficulty was to get everyone to agree. Consultants differed in the priorities to be accorded to various departments and it seems that not infrequently the attitudes of one or two Consultants could defer the start of building for months or even it was said, for years. The idea of some standardisation of hospital plans, modified only by the topography of the land and not by individual wishes was beginning to emerge as a method of speeding up building. The other continuous problem was that it was rarely possible to build on a virgin site, the problem of building a new hospital on the site of an existing one and still keeping that hospital functioning twenty-four hours a day and every day was formidable.

In the 1960's more plans for the permanent new hospital were made. We thought it would take about ten years. We were mistaken, part has been achieved — the new Maternity Unit, Casualty Department and Out-Patient Department — but sixteen years later the rest of the plan had been replaced by another one.

Meanwhile the hospital continued to function, more patients were admitted, more seen in out-patients, the casualty attendances grew and grew. Laboratory space and staff were grossly inadequate and there were increased prssures on the x-Ray Department and problems with staffing there also. Nurses were in short supply but in 1962 the General Nursing Council gave full approval to the hospital as a Training School for male and female nurses. Previously the approval granted had only been provisional but Mr J. Russell appointed Nurse Tutor for 1950 and his staff had gradually built up a small but efficient Training Department. A new School of Nursing had been opened in 1961.

In 1963 the long arguments about visiting children began to draw to a close and the medical staff with the support of the nursing staff recommended that visiting should be allowed each day from 12 noon to 7.30 p.m. Dr J.D. Andrew was appointed in July, 1963, and since then paediatric care has changed enormously and so have visiting hours. In 1964 visiting became unrestricted.

The NHS had modified and improved existing nursing and medical procedures but had not caused any really new ideas until 1964, when a decision was made that opportunity must be made within the Health Service to provide for continuing education for all qualified doctors. The old ideas that a student would learn enough during his undergraduate training to allow him to practice for the rest of his life was clearly not suitable with the great changes in knowledge in the last 20 - 30 years. It was realised that doctors ought regularly to update this knowledge and provision for this to be done in every Health District in the country was to be made.

In Bishop Auckland the BMA had held a small lecture programme — perhaps four or five a year given by distinguished Consultants, over a period of many many years and in 1950 the clinical meetings I have mentioned were started and attracted many doctors but these were not enough. A proper hospital library, a lecture theatre, and a seminar room were needed and systematic teaching programmes for junior hospital doctors, consultants and general practioners and other doctors were required. Gradually this became possible and after the new Maternity Department was built, the south end of the first floor of Block 1 and the rooms above it provided a valuable Post-Graduate Medical Centre.

The outline of the new hospital plan took shape in 1966 and was phased. The 1st phase was the building of a new Accident and Out-Patient Department and this was completed and opened in July, 1969. Thereafter phase 2 — a new Maternity Department and the provision of ancillary services — chiefly a new boiler house and engineering unit was planned. Phase 3 was to be a tall building of four or six storeys to house medical and surgical wards, operating theatres, pathology, psychiatry and long stay geriatrics. This work would also be carried out in stages. In the event the completion of the Maternity and Boiler House took longer than expected and the remainder of the plan had to be deferred.

Mr Jack Collier who had been Hospital Secretary and later Deputy Group Secretary since 1949 resigned on 14th October, 1968, to look after his sick wife. He was a quiet unassuming man who worked tirelessly and despite all the difficulties and in the early years of shortages of staff and materials, he often had to say "no" to requests, he was liked and respected by all.

As the hospital has enlarged and became much more complex it is astonishing to look back and recollect what a small staff of Administrators there were in post. It is true that they didn't deal with such a large staff, such large numbers of patients and such specialised equipment and techniques as are now required, nor, as now, were they required to deal with health in the community. Yet they had a great deal to do merely to correct the previous inertia and poor buildings, and guide and plan the present service.

The new Accident and Emergency Department was opened in July, 1969, and very soon after its completion it was put to the test by the events at Crawleyside. On 14th July, in the evening, a bus carrying old age pensioners on an outing was descending this steep bank leading down from the moors to Stanhope. Its brakes failed and it crashed. Several of the elderly were killed on the spot. The remainder were moved by ambulance to Shotley Bridge Hospital and Bishop Auckland General Hospital. A major accident plan had already been prepared a year or two previously. Because of the folds in the hills round Stanhope communication from Police to Ambulance Headquarters in Durham was difficult and some messages were relayed to a car in Bishop Auckland Hospital Grounds and then up to Stanhope. The Police and Ambulance Service did a remarkable job and some of the casualties were in Bishop Auckland within twenty minutes of being picked up on a hillside. The local people and doctors in Stanhope helped greatly. 24 patients were brought to Bishop Auckland, 3 died that night and 3 more in the next few days. Nursing and medical staff and clerical and x-ray came in — some the result of telephone messages carried out in accordance with the plan, many because they heard of the disaster and wanted to help. Everything was carried out smoothly and quickly and later the hospital was praised. One small group went almost unnoticed. These were clergymen of all denominations who arrived to help. All the patients were elderly and from the eastern part of the county, few had home telephones and in addition to their usual duties the clergy helped the police by speaking to their opposite number in the affected villages and asking them to visit the relatives to give the news. I know that without the new building we would certainly have coped — but it was made much easier by the spaciousness of the unit and this raised the morale of the staff for quite a long time.

In October, 1969, Miss Harding resigned as Matron and there were several months during which recurring temporary Matrons struggled to keep the nursing services going. Morale in the nursing staff was low and there were many shortages in all the hospitals in the Group which caused greater strain on the nursing staff. Miss D. Massey started as Matron in May, 1970. The Salmon Structure for nursing was discussed in 1970 and a start was made to implement the recommendations in June, 1971. Nursing reform was overdue but the change in the status of the ward Sister worried many. It was hoped that the new structure would reduce the "wastage" of nurses during training. At that time (1971) this was 24% at the General Hospital — almost a quarter of the nurses starting did not complete this training.

Shortage of midwives was a constant problem from 1952, restrictions of admissions were enforced from time to time and in 1972 caused temporary closure of the Princes Street Maternity Home and transfer of the patients to Bishop Auckland General Hospital.

There was a national shortage, not only of midwives but of all nurses and in December NUPE called the first one day strike and volunteers came into the hospital to help.

The need for a Consultant Physician in charge of geriatric patients was recognised and repeated attempts were made to obtain one. In 1974 none of six applicants were considered suitable for the post. This was still a shortage specialty.

Mr Luxford who had been Group Secretary since 1948 retired in May, 1974. His particular skill as I have mentioned previously was in planning. He was able to assemble small teams to redevelop a unit or a ward and managed to carry out alterations and rebuilding and many of the improvements to the hospital were due to his drive and incentive in this respect.

Reorganisation of the Health Service occurred in 1974. The Hospital Management Committee disappeared. The four Districts in County Durham came under the control of the Area Health Authority and the South West Durham District was administered by a District Management Team made up of an Administrator (Mr R.H. Wright), Treasurer, District Nursing Officer, Community Physician, General Practitioner representative and a Consultant. Before anything could happen they all had to agree — this was consensus management. They had similar opposite members on the Area Team of Officers, these latter were to monitor (one of the new fashionable words) the performance of the District Team of Officers. It was a time of great stress as many senior staff had to reapply for their job in face of open competition. It was all very unsettling and took 12 - 18 months to carry out and get people settled in their new posts. The current catchwords became "accountability upwards, delegation downwards".

One major effect of the reorganisation was that Community Services — Child Welfare and Maternity Clinics and Community Nurses together with the management of Health Centres came under the control of the District Management Team instead of the Local Authority. The other great local change was that Winterton Hospital lost its Management Committee and also came under the control of South West Durham Management Team and the Area Health Authority. There were undoubted benefits in the new arrangements but there were of course disadvantages. Both varied from District to District when seen from the perspective of the Area Health Authority and it was fairly soon realised that further organisational changes would be needed.

The Nursing Staff Changes

In 1980 nurses hours were reduced to $37^1/_2$ hours per week for basic pay but actual hours work remained 40 per week until March, 1981.

They had certainly been a change since the days of 1914 when the nurses at Holywood were contracted to do 70 hours a week. Throughout all the years since 1900 in fact there had been recurring nurses crises. Ward closures, deferment of admission and makeshift arrangements to cope with chronic nursing shortages and the high wastage of nurses in training, were needed.

The situation is still the same and reduction of hours of work and increases in salaries together with changes in conditions of work, all very necessary, have not appeared to alter the situation greatly.

In the early years Probationer nurses signed an agreement to stay three years and provided their own uniform (in most cases they got a small allowance for this). They lived in nurses homes. Married nurses in hospital were almost unknown. In Winterton in the Second World War a girl who married had to ask the Committee for permission to stay on and her contract was altered to a temporary one so that when the war ended she could be dismissed. Male nurses were found almost solely in psychiatric hospitals. The Matron was in charge of nurses, she appointed them and dismissed them. In some hospitals she decided whether a sick nurse should stay on duty or be referred to a doctor. In good hospitals she went round the wards of the hospital once or twice a every day. She spoke to patients, inspected the wards, the ward kitchens and the food, ran her fingers along shelves and leaves of the aspidistra plants to check that they were properly dusted.

She looked in all the rooms, often in the cupboards and sluices. She commented on the state of the nurse's uniform, her apron and cap, her hair and length of the dress. She kept a sharp eye on the social behaviour of her nurses and flirtations with the doctors or medical students officially did not occur!

Beneath Matron and her immediate one or two assistants was the Ward Sister. She was in charge of the ward — the patients, staff and domestic staff and all the equipment and furnishings. Woe betide her if at routine stock taking, a towel or draw sheet was missing.

Most Ward Sisters were excellent. A few were somewhat difficult and feared or disliked by their juniors. Most Sisters fought tenaciously for the patients in their care. No one came into the ward without her permission. Artisan staff, doctors and visitors had to wait at the door until she gave consent for them to enter. The patients and relatives sometimes felt a little in awe of her but after a restless night or a day when Sister was off duty, the mere sight of her duty uniform gave comfort ad reassurance and a sense of security to patients and their relatives.

However, with the shorter hours the Sister could not be present for much of the week and the introduction of the Salmon Report in 1971 changed her rôle. Change was quite inevitable but the old rôle of the Sister was diminished, Unit Nursing Officers were appointed, "delegation downwards and acting up" became the rule. Some people had the probably unworthy thought that certain staff "delegated downwards" to such a degree that they left themselves nothing to do! Many senior Sisters felt hurt at the changes, the close relationship with "her" Consultant was lessened.

In holiday period or crises a Sister would be moved up to act as Unit Nursing Officer and young Staff Nurses would move up. Sometimes it was only the senior Probationer who became Acting Nurse in Charge of the ward. Some of this had always happened, but in the past the efficient Ward Sister could always continue the administration part of her job but was able to give priority to the clinical care of the patients. Now it seemed sometimes, at least in the first few years of the administrative changes, that administration itself was more important than bedside nursing. Paperwork increased, nurses and particularly Sisters were off the wards, for conferences, study periods and various other reasons and the former lynch pin seemed to be missing.

The rapid turnover of patients made it difficult for a nurse to get to know the patients and so see the result of her nursing care as after her statutory days off when she returned all the patients were new.

Yet the increasing complexity of treatment, the demands for more precise measurement and increasing use of highly technical equipment made change in nursing organisation and practice, together with greater emphasison continuous upgrading of knowledge, absolutely essential and it is probable that the best way to solve these problems has yet to be discovered.

1977 and Onwards

In 1977 perhaps the major problem at Bishop Auckland was the shortage of Anaesthetists. It looked at one point as if the surgical side of the hospital would have to close down or to combine with Darlington to provide a service.

Fortunately these drastic steps were avoided but for several months it was uncertain whether there would be an Anaesthetist to cover surgery for the following week. This did nothing to improve morale on the surgical side but very slowly more staff were recruited and the situation improved.

Radiology was also in difficulties. There was still a national shortage of trained Consultants and we had a succession of locum Radiologists for a time.

Building, however, was continued, the new dining area complex was opened and the alterations to Block 1 finished to allow the Post-Graduate Medical Centre to open in 1977. This provided excellent facilities so that now large teaching and lecture meetings could be held and Regional and sometimes National Societies were able to come to Bishop Auckland. The hospital broadcasting service was moved to new quarters, opened in 1978. Mr C. Littlefair was Chairman of the pleasant, peaceful and useful service provided by volunteers.

The long familiar nursing shortage became worse in 1978. Durham Castle ward in the new Maternity Unit could not be used as there was a shortage of midwives. Miss Massey, the District Nursing Officer asked for the closure of a male surgical ward and on the medical side ward 3B was closed. Industrial disputes became familiar. Aycliffe Hospital laundry was severely affected and there was a shortage of clean linen in the hospitals.

In February, 1979 industrial "action" restricted admission of patients to those considered to be emergency and urgent cases. The hospitals in this District did not in fact, suffer the severe disruption seen elsewhere and on the whole there was an air of tolerance and reasonable good humour most of the time.

It was becoming clear that the new reorganisation was in need of change and another plan was proposed. It was to begin on 1st April, 1982.

Meanwhile the national oil crisis caused intense scrutiny of the use of oil, coal and electricity and some remarkable financial savings were made as staff cooperated in conserving energy.

Mr H.M. Jamison who had been on the Consultant Surgical staff since 1954 died in his sleep on 2nd August, 1980. His utter devotion to the care of his patients and his continuous efforts to improve the surgical side of the hospital were recognised, not only by the staff of the General Hospital, but by the community at large.

The Consultant Medical Staff was changing. Those appointed in the first few years of the Health Service were retiring and more Consultants were appointed. On the medical side after my retirement in 1981, Dr M.C. Bateson and Dr J.B. Walsh joined Dr G. Ismay and soon after that Dr A.J. McCulloch and Dr H. Clague joined the team. Dr Ismay retired in 1984 and when Dr Walsh left to work in Dublin, Dr R.W.G. Prescott and Dr A. Mehrzad were appointed to look after the geriatric services in addition to general medicine.

On the surgical side Mr J.G. Stephen took over after the death of Mr H.M. Jamison, and when Mr J.H. Wrigley and later Mr W. Lees retired they were succeeded by Mr C. Roberts and Mr T. Layzell.

Throughout the hospital many other staff changes occurred, some taking early retirement in the light of forthcoming changes. Miss D. Massey retired in May, 1984, and was replaced by Mr D.M. Ryan.

In 1982 Dr M.C. Bateson suggested that an appeal should be organised to raise money for a Hospital Scanner. This was considered carefully and the idea gradually took hold. In April, 1986, an appeal for £350,000 was launched. Dr D.T. Prescott became Chairman of the Appeal Committee, with Mr B. Baglee, Mr D.M. Ryan and Dr S.M. Desai to give active help. An immense amount of time and effort was put into the project. It was astonishingly successful and by 1988 at the time of writing this account almost £450,000 had been raised, much more than the original sum required.

The building to house the apparatus was erected by the Health Authority and the Scanner is due to be installed in a few weeks and will be ready for use about October, 1988. Numerous groups and individuals in the district gave great help and the press provided continuous publicity.

From April, 1982, the newly organised service took over. By now the problems faced were different from those of 1948 when the NHS began. Many diseases, tuberculosis, poliomyelitis and some of the other infectious diseases had largely disappeared. Smallpox was almost eradicated world wide. There was an increase in heart disease and cancer of the lung. More people were living longer and developing diseases of old age particularly senile dementia. Surgical techniques and resuscitation procedures and better anaesthesia had greatly altered the types of surgical cases treated. Hip and other joint replacements were common place. The supervision and management of obstetrical patients had produced dramatic falls in maternal mortality and a fall in the number of deaths in the newly born babies. The care of children and type of childrens diseases seen had changed more, babies could now be treated successfully and precise investigations carried out on these tiny babies.

Psychiatric disorders, mental subnormality, child psychiatry and the care of the physically handicapped all now pressed for attention. This meant more staff, more buildings and more money. Community Services were being developed — Community Nursing Services were now under the control of the District Health Authority.

Prevention of disease in the past had been strikingly effective. Improved sanitation, proper clean water supply, better drainage, innoculation against infectious diseases, cleaner air and better working conditions, together with improved maternity and infant care had all played a major part in the improvement of the health of the community. These of course must be continued but further improvement will be harder to achieve. This will need the active involvement of each person to improve his or her own life. Reduction in the intake of alcohol would probably save lives and improve the quality of life of vast numbers of people, reduction, or stopping smoking will halt the epidemic of cancer of the lung and prevent other illnesses. More exercise and a better diet are likely to contribute to reduction of heart and vascular disease.

In the period from 1975 onwards many changes in the hospital had occurred, a Coronary Care Unit and later an Intensive Care Unit were developed, geriatric services expanded, a travelling Psychiatric Day Hospital began at Crook and later included Bishop Auckland. The League of Friends provided £6,000 towards a minibus with a tail lift so that disabled patients could enjoy outings. The new Maternity Department, Accident and Emergency Out-Patients Department and a Day Ward had all become well established. X-ray equipment had been altered and the Pathology Department greatly enlarged. New medical and surgical techniques of investigation of patients had occurred. Changes in maternity care, the management of premature babies and the introduction of screening for cervical cancer had all taken place in the General Hospital. The care of the elderly changed, the facilities were further improved. More hostel places for the elderly were made available by the Local Authorities and later many private homes, subsidised by the DHSS sprang up. It is impossible to predict changes in the birth rate and hence provide accurate planning for maternity and infant care, but the needs for geriatric care is indeed measurable because nearly all those people now alive will become geriatric patients, though not necessarily in hospital.

For those working in hospital especially in orthopaedic and surgical wards the failure of relatives to take their elderly patients home gives rise to the feeling that sons and daughters do not want their parents. Occasionally this is true but more often it is not, and the physical conditions just do not permit the younger relations to cope with the elderly. Furthermore a few elderly people have been so awkward and demanding that they have managed almost totally to destroy the marriages of the younger members of the family. A few old people have neglected or ill treated their families throughout life and it is hard to see why such young people should be required to help their aged parents.

However, the picture seen in hospital is not representative. I was able to see many elderly people looked after by their relatives. It was common to see a daughter looking after her husband and two or three children, travel sometimes by one or two journeys to see her father or mother several times a week, to do the washing, shopping or housework. Such help in itself is not assisted, when at holiday times, some other relative, often from a great distance arrives and insists "something must be done". This usually means — by someone else. All doctors are familiar with the "distant relative syndrome" and are used to being called on Christmas Eve, Christmas Day or the New Year and Easter holidays. I was involved in this way every Christmas without exception for over thirty years. Fortunately nowadays better community services, short term care admissions to hospital or hostels together with day units can all help to reduce the burdens on the relatives and in many cases improve the health of the elderly. Much more needs to be done and Chiropodists and Physiotherapists especially, are still in short supply. Probably only about five per cent of elderly patients are in long term hospital care, but as more people are living to old age that number may rise.

The new organisation in 1982 reinstated the District Management Committee, but it was now called the District Health Authority. The District Management Team was altered a little and everyone assumed a new title. There was now in post, a Unit General Manager, Director of Finance, Director of Midwifery Services, Unit Management Groups, a District Planning Team, to mention but a few. These were always referred to by their initials so that when I came to read the Minutes I felt the need of a reference book of initials. It was perhaps remarkable that despite all these changes normal control of the hospital and community services continued.

The language used in the Minutes had changed, the clear simple words of the early Minutes usually hand written were replaced by repeated initials. The old term Matron and Hospital Secretary had gone. The former Assistant Chief Nurse at the General Hospital became the Senior Nursing Officer, then in succession, Divisional Nursing Officer, Director of Nursing Services, and now is dignified by the title Patient Services Manager. Fortunately when I met him recently he seemed much the same person as usual, carrying out his duties quietly and with a sense of humour and not overwhelmed by the sonority of his title.

Yet despite some progress there were disadvantages. The Minutes become voluminous, the few sheets of some years ago now became at least twenty or thirty. The words strategy, planning, resources, projections and other such terms appeared frequently so that the odd rare reference to a patient was welcome and reminded me that it was a Health Service that was being considered.

Some things, as usual in a large organisation, with many sub-sections got out of proportion. One sub-committee spent some months considering the problem of SHARPS. The word was always written in capital letters and I did not at first know what it meant. The question considered was indeed serious — the real possibility that anyone handling used needles from syringes and other sharp items of equipment might accidentally prick themselves and become infected, sometimes with a possibly fatal disease. A code of practice had long been in force in the hospitals to reduce such a risk. Now, however, a General Practitioner wrote to ask what action the hospital could take to help him with the problem of disposing of such used items. The sub-committee considered the matter and made investigations. A report was received detailing the build and mechanics of the modern refuse collection vehicle and the crushing equipment used, collecting boxes, points of collection, staffing needs, and costs were considered. Finally a reply was sent to the wrong doctor in the wrong village, and the recipient denied all knowledge of the correspondence. Meanwhile the original General Practitioner who had posed the question, had retired from General Practice. It was not until Mr D.M. Ryan became General Manager and the problem was put before him that he solved it in less than ten minutes.

In the 1982 reorganisation the District Management Team became the District Policy Review Group but still consensus of all the members was needed. Later the title was again changed to District Management Board. Mr D.M. Ryan was made District General Manager and the duties of each of the senior officials clearly defined.

The voluminous Minutes began to shrink, decisions were made more quickly and more clearly.

Planning for the future continues but not, as so often in the past, by pious expressions that this or that was needed, but by clearly describing the reasons, needs and consequences, together with the staffing and financial implications of any proposed action. This seems to be a welcome reform and should bode well for the future.

It is very difficult to sum up the history and achievements of the hospitals over the last hundred years. The changing social conditions, the newer types of diseases and the greater variety of powerful methods of treatment, together with an immense increase in investigation in diagnosis and management, have all raised the expectations of the community. All these factors continue and will continue to change. What we regard as necessary now in 1988 will almost certainly be different in twenty years time. Planning for the Health Service is a difficult art, not a science. Much of hospital care has been to try to improve the quality of life of the patient. Sometimes it has failed totally to do so. At times it has become possible to cure the patient. It seems to me, however, that prevention of diseases and injury is still the chief goal. There will, however, always be a need for the care and treatment of the sick and the hospitals of South West Durham mentioned in this account will play an increasing role in fullfilling this need.

1988

As can be deduced from the account so far there have been immense changes since the start of the National Health Service.

Recently I was able to see two of them within a few days. The childrens ward together with the section of the Bishop Auckland Health Centre devoted to community paediatrics arranged an open day and a few days later the newly installed scanner was open to view.

The childrens' ward was completely rebuilt at a cost of about £300,000 and reopened in 1985. Dr Andrew retired in 1987 and Dr Cottrell, Dr Lamb and Dr Jones now run the unit and community paediatrics.

When I saw the new ward and recalled the first ward that was used for children in 1950 the change was remarkable. Gone was the bare long ward with two coke stoves and a line of beds on each side. Then there were no side wards, no decoration on the walls, and very few toys in evidence. Most of the children were over the age of three — usually 7 - 14 and often suffering from long term illnesses — rheumatic fever, St. Vitus dance, heart diseases, tuberculosis in its various forms, appendicitis and injuries. Most children remained largely in bed and the risk of infection brought in from outside was always present. I did not admit babies under the age of three years as we had no proper isolation facilities. Instead I saw babies on the day the request was made (including weekends) and either arranged treatment at home or if hospital admission was needed, rang up the Royal Victoria Infirmary or Newcastle General Hospital, where by prior arrangement with Professor Spence or Dr George Davison and his colleagues, the baby would immediately be admitted. This arrangement lasted for some three years until we got some side ward accommodation.

Now the ward doesn't look like an ordinary ward. There is a large reception counter in the middle, cots and beds are scattered about, the unit is full of drawings and pictures, often made by the children, toys of all sizes and types abound, there is an air of normal untidiness associated with children, white coated doctors are not seen — most are casually dressed. It reminds me that Professor Spence used to say that a true paediatrician had baggy knees to his trousers as he always knelt down to examine his small patients! There is a room fitted up as a school room with a teacher, books and writing materials are in abundance and a computer is available. The atmosphere is informal and pleasant. There are rooms in which a parent can sleep while the child is in hospital. Relatives of the children are welcome and take part in the nursing care. Should a child have to go to the operating theatre or elsewhere he can be carried on Thomas the Tank Engine.

More babies are admitted and many of the older diseases mentioned have largely gone. The equipment is sophisticated, and usually small, in keeping with the size of the patients and an astonishing degree of accuracy in diagnosis and observation of the children is now possible throughout the whole 24 hours.

Outside the ward is a play area. The Lions Club paid for the equipment.

No one entering this unit has any doubt that this is a childrens ward — not just another ward in a general hospital. Most of the children nowadays can be managed at home or as hospital out-patients and those who are admitted, are in hospital for the shortest possible time. During their stay, most will get up, play or attend the school as they feel able to do.

The other change concerned the scanner. I was shown around in one of the evening inspection times together with many others. The immaculate new building, the gleaming, sophisticated, smooth machinery and the marvellously clear images produced made me quite envious. As I write I happen to have alongside me the list of basic equipment that I had to order when the medical wards were starting up in 1950 — simple items like thermometers, stethoscopes, opthalmoscopes, tape measures and weighing machines. The most elaborate was a heavy portable electrocardiogram powered by large accumulators and which cost about £400. The whole cost of all the equipment was under £1,000 and I recall going to the Senior Administrative Medical Officer to ask for an extra allocation of money to start up the ward. The scanner was provided by the generosity and hard work of innumerable people in South West Durham and cost £350,000. The hospital authorities provided the building.

Some £450,000 was raised so the extra sum will pay the running costs for the first year.

Although I have mentioned the childrens' ward and scanner because of the coincidence of the opening days, almost any section of the hospital can show equally remarkable changes so that though some of the external aspects of the building are not greatly altered, inside all is different.

Yet the most impressive change of all, was psychological. The people of the community were frightened and suspicious of the hospital in 1950. Now they work gladly and continuously for it, and though no one likes being a patient, are glad to use the casualty, out-patient and in-patient services. It has become their hospital, an essential part of the community of South West Durham. This is not the picture of a service in terminal decline, as some would have us believe.

The Hospitals in Upper Weardale and the Early Days of Treatment of Tuberculosis

Although tuberculosis was not yet a notifiable disease in the regulations of 1899, it was a very common illness. It chiefly affected children and young adults and many people died, sometimes of severe bleeding from the lung, sometimes from tuberculous meningitis which was then invariably fatal. Not only did the germ attack the lungs — producing "consumption" as it was often called but glands, bones, joints and abdominal organs were often affected.

In the last few years of the last century it was widely believed that fresh air, good food and a combination of rest and graduated exercises could cure some patients and improve many others. No curative drug treatments for the disease were known.

Dr William Robinson is well described by Dr A.J.A. Ferguson in his section of this book. Dr Robinson was always interested in tuberculosis as he had seen a great deal of this disease while looking after lead miners in Weardale. In 1898 he called a meeting, which was held in the Town Hall at Sunderland and that night formed the Sunderland and District Branch of the Society for the Prevention and Care of Consumption in County Durham.

Within one year money had been raised, committees formed, and in August, 1899, Dr Robinson showed lantern slides of possible sites in the neighbourhood of Stanhope, where he thought that a hospital for tuberculosis patients could be established. The ten members of the Executive Committee thought that the Wear Valley at Stanhope "offered special facilities, including water power to produce electric power, drinking water is readily accessible and walks are sheltered from the wind by woods. The eastern side of the stream seems drier and more suitable than the western". Three sites were inspected and one was selected on which to build. As this would take time the Committee agreed to try to rent a building for up to five years while erecting the new one. They thought an ordinary house, with grounds large enough in which to erect up to ten wooden chalets as bedrooms would suffice. The aim was eventually to provide some forty beds. The Committee thought that patients would pay say 30/- per week. The Ecclesiastical Commissioners heard of the search for a house and offered the Committee the lease of Horn Hall for temporary use at £40 per year. In addition there were some nine acres of land which the Committee could have as a permanent site for 999 years at £5 per year.

Mr Mews the tenant of the Hall was leaving. The Committee accepted the tenancy of Horn Hall and paid Mr and Mrs Mews £10 so that he would leave earlier than the expiry of his tenancy. Horn Hall was thought to be about 200 years old.

Alterations were made to the Hall and a new temporary external dining room was added.

Rules were drawn up to govern the conduct of patients and staff based on those used in other sanatoria. The first patients were admitted on 15th May, 1900, and the Hall was officially opened by Lord Barnard on 9th June, 1900, some twenty months after the inaugural meeting in the Sunderland Town Hall. Miss Rawlings, a Deaconess, with the permission of the Bishop of Durham, was appointed Matron, Dr Chiddell was appointed Medical Superintendent but his health broke down soon after his appointment in January, 1900, and he had to withdraw before patients were admitted. Hence Dr John Gray a Practitioner in Wolsingham was appointed in a temporary capacity at a fee of two guineas a week.

Miss Rawlings wanted more staff and as they did not materialise she resigned and Miss McWilliam was appointed at £35 per year. There were twelve beds for patients but soon after the opening the Committee decided to build a new wing so that twenty patients could be admitted. A new lease — a "repairing lease" at £35 per year for 80 years was negotiated with the Ecclesiastical Commissioners. The Committee would do all internal and external repairs.

By 1902 the new wing was in use, 29 patients were in the hospital and the Matron's salary was increased to £48 per year. The septic tank was working well, Sunderland Corporation supported two beds by paying £75 per year and other Local Authorities were considering doing the same. Industrial firms also subscribed and workmen in the large firms allowed 2d or 3d per quarter to be deducted from their wages to help to maintain Horn Hall. Workmen governors were nominated and served on the Management Committee.

By 1905 both men and women were accepted as patients and there were 45 in all. After only one year — in 1901 — it was decided to sell the piggery — the smell and close proximity to the Hall were too much and the household refuse formerly given to the pigs was now to be sold.

The Committee took a keen interest in the treatment of the patients, Dr Gray still had two guineas a week but he also now received 1/- per week for each occupied bed beyond the original twelve beds. He provided the necessary drugs as part of his contract. In 1906 the Committee suggested through the Chairman — Dr Robinson — that Dr Gray should use the recently introduced tuberculin treatment. Dr Robinson gave meticulous information on how to administer the remedy, how and where to purchase it, the exact dosage and frequency and the type of case best suited for the treatment. He also included reference in the current literature concerning the treatment. I do not think that present day Management Committees, even with medical members would attempt this.

By 1907 the need for more beds was apparent and a new sanatorium was sought. Mr Roddam was asked if he was prepared to sell Newtown House in Stanhope but he declined. Advertisements were put in the local press inviting the sale of a suitable house or land for use as a sanatorium, and in October, 1908, Leazes House, Wolsingham (which had been built before 1839) had been offered. The Committee inspected the house and agreed to buy it. It was to provide 28 beds for patients and five for resident staff. The large field which came with the house was to be let.

Nurse Swinburn was appointed Matron 1st February, 1909, at £40 per year and Dr Menzies of Wolsingham was made Medical Officer at £5 per occupied bed (but not more than £120 per year), and he was to provide all necessary drugs. Lord Barnard officially opened Leazes House on 1st May, 1909, and twenty patients were resident by 31st May.

In 1912 the Clerk to the Durham County Council wrote to the Committee offering to take over Leazes and Horn Hall Sanatoria. The Committee agreed to negotiate on the matter but nothing more was mentioned in the Minutes thereafter and in 1913 the County Council, as will be seen later bought Holywood Hall for use as a sanatorium.

In 1913 a curious episode occurred. Leazes House had been an active sanatorium for four years when a Mr Gillespie approached the Committee asking if his unnamed client, could purchase the building to reconvert it into a private house. He offered £3,000. The Executive Committee thought this was not enough but by June the offer was raised to £3,250 and was accepted. However, at the Annual Court of Governors later in the same month it was unanimously agreed to not go ahead with the sale. The members at both meetings were almost identical but no mention of the discussions which took place or who actually voted for, or against the sale in the first place, is recorded. Leazes Hall therefore continued as a sanatorium.

In 1916, the War was in progress and the Committee agreed to insure both Horn Hall and Leazes against air raids.

As often happens in a closed community, friction occurred from time to time. In July, 1909, the patients at Horn Hall sent a petition to the Committee of Management. They objected to paying 30/- a week for their accomodation and treatment and at the same time being required to perform work e.g. washing up (many, of course did not pay as they were supported by their council or works). The Committee were not sympathetic and replied "That the patients should do work in a sanatorium is now a recognised and valuable adjunct to treatment and prevents the development of indolence. It is for the Medical Superintendent to select the patients fit for work and the kind of work suitable for each. Should any disobey, he (the Medical Superintendent), must act according to the rules of the institution. In the Kings Sanatorium each patient who can, must work three hours a day though the patient pays £3.3.0 per week. There is no reason why the Medical Officer should fail where these succeed in this matter".

Children were admitted in 1924 — ten boys to Horn Hall at a cost of 37/6 per week and nine to Leazes and the following year Dr J.F. McConchie was made deputy to Dr Menzies at Leazes. By 1927 a new recreation hall was built at Horn Hall to provide for games and Billiards, by then there were 29 adults and 18 children in Horn Hall and 22 Female and 9 children in Leazes.

In Horn Hall the boys had tea and supper combined at 5 p.m. and bread and dripping or butter at 7 p.m. and had to be in bed at 7.30 p.m.

About the same time the Committee tried to insist that wholemeal bread was used at both sanatoria. They told the Matrons to buy it at Hindhaughs or Allisons. Whether it was used at Horn Hall is not recorded. At Leazes, however, the Minutes on several occasions state that Matron is to be reminded about the need to use wholemeal bread. This was from 1927 to about 1931.

The education of the children posed problems. A teacher would cost money and this would increase the weekly charge per patient. Local Authorities — who now paid for most of the patients — were already objecting to the present cost. The Ministry of Education said they would only consent to the appointment of a teacher if the Local Authorities would pay. There was stalemate. However the Committee agreed to accept a Mr McClaren as a patient without payment, provided he would give instruction at Horn Hall, to those boys approved by Dr Gray.

Clothing the children also caused difficulty and in 1928 the Committee ordered that the parents were to be asked first to provide the clothing, if that failed then the Local Authorities should be approached, but if neither parties were able to supply the clothing, then Matron would obtain what was necessary and the Committee would pay.

Two uncertificated teachers were appointed — Miss Fairless at Horn Hall (£141 per yer) and Miss Salton at Leazes (£99 per year). Desks, furniture and books were provided and the cost for women and children was increased from 5/- per day at Leazes and the same for the boys at Horn Hall. Charges for the men were not raised.

A small garden was provided for the boys at each institution. A school library linked to Durham County Council Library was started. At Horn Hall it was ordered that the stables were to be thoroughly cleaned and whitewashed, the stable yard and coach house were to be kept in a perfectly clean condition, and that no refuse was to be allowed to accumulate where the children had swings. In December Miss Walton at Leazes complained that she and the children were suffering from the cold, and asked for a stove. The school was held in an open chalet. The Committee reluctantly agreed that a stove formerly used in the surgery should be tried as an experiment.

The Board of Education agreed the proposed time tables for the schools, provided that the first ten minutes of the arithmetic period should be devoted to breathing and physical exercises. By the end of 1929 there were 29 boys in school at Horn Hall and 13 in Leazes.

Dr Chapman of the Ministry of Health inspected Leazes and recommended that extra bathrooms be provided, together with other changes to allow four more children to be admitted and replace three women. However, the prudent Committee replied that all the children had their baths under proper supervision before 7 p.m. and the women had the use of the baths after that. However, new plans for extensions were drawn up.

On 17th September, 1930, Dr John Gray died suddenly. He had been Medical Superintendent at Horn Hall for 30 years and of Leazes also for the last four years. Dr O'Hara was made Acting Medical Superintendent.

Quite soon the duties of the Superintendent of each sanatorium were more clearly defined and the relations between the two outlined. Now there was to be a visiting Medical Superintendent to oversee both sanatoria, and for this post Dr Geoffrey Robinson, son of Dr William Robinson was appointed. He was to visit the hospitals on two set days per month, supervise and direct the treatment in conjunction with the Medical Officers and receive £240 per year. Dr O'Hara became Medical Officer to Horn Hall and Dr J.F. McConchie to Leazes from 1st December, 1930.

Other santatoria had appeared in the North of England, especially Holywood Hall at Wolsingham and there was competition to reduce costs. Leazes and Horn Hall reduced their charges to 30/- per week. There was, however, no shortage of patients but there was shortage of money to pay for them.

Dr Geoffrey Robinson reported on his attendance at the 1932 Conference of the National Association for the Prevention of Tuberculosis and gave details of the discussions. He said that the death rate from tuberculosis was falling but still remained high between the ages of 15 and 25, indeed the rate had risen between those ages. Various factors thought to be responsible were named, amongst them were:- Votes for women and flappers, the wearing of artificial silk instead of red flannel or pink flanelette, late hours at dances or cinemas and other entertainments, cocktails, hurried insufficient and unsuitable meals, long and tiring journeys to and from work, indoor employment in works and offices, especially underground with rooms ill lit all day by artificial light when girls worked elbow to elbow and row upon row. Two other causes operated on all ages — smokey dirty atmosphere by burning raw coal in open fireplaces, "which screens off ultra violet light which helps to manufacture disease protecting vitamins within the body", and personal lack of cleanliness and dirt in the streets.

The first apparatus for the induction of the new treatment of artificial pneumothorax was bought in 1935 for £10 and Dr O'Hara went to the Brompton Hospital in London for four days to learn the technique but it was nearly six months later before he found a patient thought to be suitable for that treatment.

The Committee considered nurses accommodation in both sanatoria in 1937. They admitted that the conditions were poor and grim. Horn Hall, they said did not lend itself to extensive change. (As can be seen today a wall inside is about two feet thick). Leazes was better being brighter and more cheery with more evidence of forethought and consideration. The Committee felt that "the main building of Horn Hall does the Committee no credit, the rooms for nurses lacked the homely touch and were cold and drab". Improvements were made but the structure of the building prevented major changes.

In 1938 the Committee reported on the recreation of the patients. Walks took place between 9.30 and 11 a.m. and from 2.30 to 4 p.m. Billiards was played in the recreation hall but very few patients were fit enough to play table tennis. Card games and whist drives were common. No gambling was allowed. Croquet was played but new balls were needed. There was an excellent library.

The boys did gardening, went for walks, played cricket, read and had private games. The wireless was now available, a gramophone also and there was a piano and of course the school. Religious services were held regularly.

One gets the impression when reading the Minutes at this time that the Committee was becoming elderly and youthful replacements not coming forward. Much of the original zest had gone. Dr William Robinson was still the mainspring. The Committee decided not to make any changes in the running of the sanatoria, including the hours of duty of the staff. There was not guarantee that the beds would be occupied in the near future. This was around the time of the Munich crisis. In 1935 Dr O'Hara started taking x-rays and in September five adults and three children had x-rays and the same number had radioscopic exams. (We would call it screening now i.e. no film was made and the doctor reported on what he saw when looking at the screen). Six patients from Leazes were also x-rayed.

Preparation for War in 1938 were made. The hospitals were warned that they might be taken over and the existing patients discharged and South Shields, Gateshead and West Hartlepool Councils were told that they may be required to take back their patients. Surgical treatment of pulmonary tuberculosis was being tried elsewhere but Dr William Robinson reported that in his view the open air treatment had revoluntionised all hospital treatment and also had affected the ordinary housing and life of the people whereas surgical treatment had not come up to expectations.

A suggestion was made that both Leazes and Horn Hall should become open air schools for the children of families suffering from pulmonary tuberculosis with 40 girls at Leazes and 50 boys at Horn Hall. Negotiations with interested Committees were started but were overtaken by the start of the 1939 War when many patients were discharged until only twelve remained at Horn Hall and seven at Leazes.

In 1940 Dr J.F. McConchie began, at his own expense, to try the new gold injection treatment for certain cases of tuberculosis at Leazes. The Committee agreed to reimburse him and awarded him £5. In response to the Government appeal the Committee sent all their supply of aluminium hot water bottles and all aluminium equipment that they could spare. Also in the same year Dr William Robinson failed to attend the annual Court of Governors. This was the first time he was absent for 40 years.

Some years ago, I recall being told by a former Night Sister at Horn Hall of her duties.She had to try to protect the patients in the riverside two storey block from the weather. The upper storey housed most of the patients chiefly in single rooms. The windows overlooked the river but as the bed head was under the window the patients all looked away from the river. The door entering the cubicles from the corridor which ran the length of the block on the side away from the river, were half doors up to waist height and in two halves so that when both halves were open a bed or trolley could go through. The outside corridor had a wooden rail on its outer side and the floor of the corridor was wooden planks separated by a few inches between each plank to maintain continuous ventilation. There was a roof over the corridor but no wall on the side away from the building — just the wooden rails. The windows of the cubicles were kept open and no heating was provided. Fresh air was the main stay of treatment. During windy, wet and especially snowy weather, Sister had to go round with heavy rubber sheets to cover the bed clothes to keep out the rain and snow and also she had to provide a continuous supply of hot water bottles. The journey from the main hall to the riverside block was of course through the open air.

For those who have worked in Horn Hall — as I have — the buildings are almost totally unsuitable for their purpose and always have been despite alterations. It is a constant reminder that buildings alone do not make a hospital, indeed are never the most important part. It is the spirit and care provided by the staff despite the difficult surroundings that matter. Fortunately Horn Hall has been well served in this respect and the loyal service of the nursing and domestic staff under physical difficulties deserves great praise.

Dr William Robinson died while on holiday at Newton Hotel, Stanhope, on the 9th December, 1940, at the age of 81. He was a remarkable man and the driving force for many years in the management of the two sanatoria. His academic career has been mentioned by Dr Ferguson and was distinguished. In October, 1934, on the occasion of the centenary celebrations of the College of Medicine in Newcastle he was awarded the rare distinction of a honorary degree of Doctorate of Surgery, by the University of Durham.

During the War London County Council sent civilians suffering from tuberculosis to both sanatoria. Poole Sanatorium on Teesside was partially opened in 1942 and Sunderland and South Shields began to give up using Leazes Hospital and in the next year also ceased to use Horn Hall.

An X-Ray set was at last obtained in 1942 and installed at Leazes. The electricity supply had previously been unsuitable for an X-Ray Unit. Dr J.F. McConchie received £40 per annum for using the new apparatus and began to use artificial pneumothorax treatment. In October, 1943 the Committee, to overcome the shortage of fat in the diet of the patients ordered a supply of malt at 42/- per 28 lb.

Durham County Council still used beds at both sanatoria and in 1944 it was agreed to restrict the use by the London County Council of the beds to allow Durham priority. 10 beds at Horn Hall and 12 at Leazes were allowed for the London patients though they had asked for almost twice those numbers.

After the war ended Messrs. Milburn, the Sunderland Architects at the request of the Ministry of Health, drew plans for extensive rebuilding of both hospitals. Children were still admitted in 1946 but it was understood they would soon be withdrawn. No action was taken over these new plans because the new NHS was to start in 1948. In October, 1947, the Committee received final notice that Horn Hall and Leazes would be taken over by the new NHS. The Committee agreed that there was nothing that could be done in this matter and in November, 1947, the last Annual General Meeting of the Committee was held. There were only seven people present, the Chairman and Secretary were both absent due to illness.

Dr O'Hara resigned in 1948 as he was leaving his practice and recommended Dr D. Thomson O.B.E. as his successor and this was approved. Dr J.F. McConchie was made Senior Medical Officer over both sanatoria and responsible for pneumothorax treatment and his son James became his Assistant Medical Officer at Leazes. The existing Medical Superintendent Dr Geoffrey Robinson continued as before.

The last Minutes of the Committee were written on 16th June, 1948. There would be a Meeting of the Annual Court of Governors that year. The Secretary was asked to prepare an Annual Report but it was recognised that there would be considerable difficulties in getting it printed in a reasonable time and I have not been able to find any such report.

Thus the Committee formed with such enthusiasm and drive at Sunderland in 1898 came to a quiet end, and though I feel that the members would be saddened I also believe that they may have felt a sense of relief.

Under the new management the two sanatoria continued to care for patients with tuberculosis and were now controlled by South West Durham Hospital Management Committee and the Newcastle Regional Hospital Board. At the time of transfer Horn Hall had 44 beds and Leazes 33 beds.

Mr Norman Richards, the Chief Clerk at Holywood Hall Hospital, Wolsingham, was appointed Administrative Assistant, in charge of Horn Hall, Leazes, Holywood Hall and the Weardale Isolation Hospital.

On the 15th May, 1950, Horn Hall celebrated its 50th anniversary as a sanatorium.

Nationally the incidence of tuberculosis had been slowly falling but there were still long waiting lists at the sanatoria for treatment. In 1948, streptomycin was discovered. Research on the use of this drug was intensive and Horn Hall, Leazes and Holywood Hall all took part in systematic research organised by a National Committee. By 1957 the number of patients was falling quickly and wards were being shut and Physicians who had spent their life look after tuberculosis patients were becoming redundant. Already in 1955 the tuberculosis ward at Homelands Hospital, Crook — used only for advanced cases — was closed and in 1956 the Regional Hospital Board considered closing Horn Hall completely.

Holywood Hall Hospital

The third hospital in Weardale — the largest — was Holywood Hall which was built by Charles Atwood, the founder of the steel works at Tudhoe in 1864 as his home. Subsequently it was owned by the Misses Rogerson and then by Mr Vickers from whom it was bought by Durham County Council in 1913.

Soon after the house was taken over by the Council, 100 roses were ordered, and they were not to cost more than six pence each. They were to replace existing old roses which were unfit to be moved and replanted following alterations to the building.

It was opened in 1914 for 25 patients and was to be the main sanatorium for patients in County Durham at that time. A Medical Superintendent, Matron, one Sister, one Staff Nurse, two Probationer Nurses and a Cook, a Kitchen Maid and three Housemaids were appointed.

The Matron and Medical Superintendent had no fixed hours but were resident in the Hall. The remaining nurses and domestic staff were to work 70 hours a week. The Sister received £40 per year and had three weeks holiday. The youngest Housemaid — a girl of about 16 years worked 70 hours a week, received £13 a year and had 10 days holiday a year.

With the Hall, came the surrounding land. This was extensive and included Baal Hill Farm which was rented to a local farmer. The water supply was from a spring in the hillside which was piped into a storage tank. Wolsingham District Council refused to accept sewage from Holywood Hall and suggested that the hospital should provide its own scheme within the grounds.

Despite the War, plans to extend the facilities were made and in 1915 a new pavilion for patients was built and a house erected for the Medical Superintendent. The Hall continued to house some patients and also was the dining accommodation for all the patients and, of course, the staff also lived in it. Electric light was installed via a generating plant run on oil. There was a supply of accumulators to act as a reserve. The total number of lights to be provided was expected to be 640 but initially only 175 were to be wired up.

Only patients expected to recover were to be admitted and by the end of 1916 further shelters had been erected — mainly open fronted huts so that there were 40 patients in the new pavilion, 24 in the permanent shelters and 30 children were housed in the Hall itself — the total being 94, and further buildings were to be erected. Those living in the Hall used temporary mobile earth closets. The permanent shelters were made of wood and the Committee considered that these "only rarely cause the patients serious inconveniences" and that more protection against rain could be provided at small cost. The chief "treatment", of course, in those days, consisted in ample fresh air, good food and graduated rest and exercise, possibly in that order.

A teacher was appointed for the children in 1916 and the nursing staff increased to 10 (excluding Matron) to look after 94 patients. Gradually the buildings increased in number and from 1919 huts from the Stanhope Prisoner of War Camp or from Rosehill were bought, and in all 10 huts were eventually moved to Holywood Hall. Some of these continued to be in use until the hospital was closed in 1986.

It was suggested that both men and women should be admitted in 1919 — at present only men were admitted. The Medical Superintendent rejected the idea. He wrote to the Committee, "the narrow ground $1^1/_2$ miles long on hilly ground and wooded on one side made supervision difficult. The effect of mixing is unquieting and undesirable from the point of view of treatment".

More huts from disused camps were bought in 1920 and 1921, by 1927 some 210 beds were in use.

As had been the case for a short time at Horn Hall a piggery was introduced and the Minutes of the Committee from 1915 often refer to the death of a pig and sometimes offer remarkable causes of death. One patient was employed as the pig keeper and paid 15/- per week.

By 1929 the water supply was inadequate. Two more springs were inspected but it was agreed to try to extend the supply given by Durham County Water Board which up to now had only been used as an emergency supply and then only to the Hall itself. The problem was cost. The spring water was free and the pipes and storage tanks were provided whereas the Water Board charged for their water. In the same year the electricity plant was causing problems and the supply was then obtained from the Cleveland and Durham County Electrical Power Company.

A lot of time was spent considering whether the sanatorium and its grounds should be converted to a village settlement like Papworth in Cambridgeshire with sheltered accommodation and workshops. After discussions lasting nearly two years, it was decided that as the prospects for work in the county as a whole were so poor, that sheltered workshops would not be viable but all through the 1930's the suggestion kept reappearing.

Artificial pneumothorax treatment was begun in 1932 and about the same time gold injections were tried and these were continued until the 1940's. Surgery was considered and in 1935 tenders were invited from Consultant Surgeons to provide costs for consultations, minor operation fees, and a post operative fee. Two Surgeons from Newcastle put in tenders and though they differed under the three headings, the cheapest was that of Mr George Mason and he was appointed. Prior to that, in 1928 Mr H.M. Johnston, a Consultant Surgeon at the Royal Victoria Infirmary had acted as visiting Surgeon to Holywood and was paid for each visit. In 1937 he resigned and was replaced by Mr F.C. Pybus who transferred occasional patients to the Royal Victoria Infirmary to carry out the operation of thoracoplasty — a major operation. Mr Mason was to do minor surgery at Holywood Hall itself and was paid an annual salary and a new operating theatre and x-ray department was opened in 1937. Up to 1946 patients with surgical tuberculosis — of bones and joints chiefly,were admitted but then this practice ceased and only chest — pulmonary tuberculosis — patients were admitted.

There was always a nursing shortage but by 1947 a ward had to be shut because there were too few nurses and only 147 out of 184 beds could be used and there was a large waiting list for admission. It was decided to admit only very early cases — chiefly those picked up by the new technique of mass minature radiography. In the same year Mr Mason took over the patients needing thorocoplasty and admitted them to his wards at Shotley Bridge Hospital.

The introduction of streptomycin in 1948 accelerated the decline in the number of cases of tuberculosis and slowly other drugs were added, each of which increased the likelihood of cure or at least making the patient non infectious which of course reduced the risk to others, especially children, in the homes of patients. Milk born tuberculosis, usually due to milk from tuberculous cattle was disappearing because of the development of herds free from tuberculosis.

Holywood Hall played a full part in the nationally organised clinical trials of these new drugs so that the combined experience of all doctors treating tuberculosis could be used. This quickened the discovery of the most effective way of using these drugs. A few national clinical trials of other drugs had been carried out previously for other diseases, but this was one of the biggest and because of the chronicity of the disease, one of the most difficult to organise and evaluate. It was undoubtedly one of the great successes of the new NHS that such trials could be organised and now they are fairly commonplace. This was an exciting time for doctors, patients and staff and in addition the newer surgical techniques carried out by Mr Mason and Mr Barnsley at Holywood also raised morale and gave renewed hope to the patients.

Whenever I visited Holywood Hall, especially in winter, I felt the patients must be fairly fit and strong. On a cold winter morning, with snow and ice on the paths and a slope upwards from the Hall to the wards of about thirty degrees it was quite a hard climb. The staff and patients did this several times a day.

Dr J.W. Gray having been Medical Superintendent over 25 years retired in 1951. He was succeeded by Dr Peter Parkinson. He took over at a time of financial crisis in the Health Service. As far as Holywood went this caused a halt to the reinstatement of 25 beds which had been out of use while upgrading of the wards occurred. Later in the same year the Regional Health Authority suggested that women patients should be admitted in addition to the men. This time there were no objections and in April, 1952, one ward of 37 beds was used for females. This was the first time since the hospital opened that women had been patients. Also in the same year it was agreed that provided the water supply to the hospital via the springs, could be secured, that Baal Hill Farm should be sold. The expenditure on the farm exceeded income by £270 in each of the last three years. The farmer would continue to supply the hospital with tuberculin tested milk. Durham County Council took over the moorland springs and the existing pipes and storage tanks and the necessary area of land.

More new drugs had been developed and now it was possible to render the patient non infectious within a few weeks. It began to be safe to discharge the patient early to continue his drugs at home. Formerly a stay in hospital of one or two years had been fairly common — now only a few weeks were needed. Many did not need admission at all and could be treated as outpatients. As a result waiting lists fell and beds became empty.

In 1954 Dr Parkinson suddenly collapsed and died. He had during the short time of his tenure effected many changes in the running of the hospital and had seen the drastic changes due to drug therapy. Later in the year Dr J.S. Law became Superintendent.

By 1957 the decline of the disease led to the centralisation of all the cases in South West Durham at Holywood. The beds at Tindale Crescent Hospital and Homelands Hospital used for tuberculosis were shut in 1955 and refills of artificial pneumothorax carried out on out-patients at the Lady Eden ceased. Indeed that form of treatment started in this area in 1935 was almost vanishing. It was practised all over the country but there was never any proof that it was effective. It was widely assumed to be so, but the techniques of evaluating new treatment for chronic fluctuating diseases had not then been developed whereas now such a scheme was in place to scrutinise the value of streptomycin and now it was possible to quantify the results quite precisely.

At last the piggery started in 1915, was discontinued in 1961 — the profit had been declining and the previous yeard had only made £45.

Surgery for pulmonary tuberculosis ceased at Holywood in 1963 and the few operations needed were carried out at Shotley Bridge Chest Unit. The vacant operating theatre could not be used by the Bishop Auckland Surgeons because of the shortage of Anaesthetists. Accordingly it was used once a week for minor surgical cases transferred from the waiting list of Newcastle General Hospital and a Surgeon from Hexham, or the General Hospital, at Newcastle came across with an Anaesthetist to do the operation. The patients stayed in the surgical wards a few days in Wolsingham and in addition post operative patients from Newcastle General Hospital were transferred to Holywood to recuperate. Some 10 beds were used in this way and Dr James L. McConchie looked after these patients.

In November, 1964, the last two cases of pulmonary tuberculosis remaining in Holywood Hall were transferred to Maiden Law Hospital. Thus 50 years after opening for the treatment of tuberculosis that era ended.

Dr Law now had sessions at Dryburn and Bishop Auckland for the management of other diseases of the chest and Dr Clark assisted him. Non-Tuberculosis chest diseases were admitted to Holywood Hall but the old office of Medical Superintendent was discontinued in 1963.

Most of the beds at Holywood were now empty and the Regional Health Authority agreed that they should be used to relieve the severe overcrowding at Winterton Hospital. There were many patients who had lived for years in Winterton and had no contact with any relatives and had no visitors. They did not need active therapy and were mainly elderly. By March, 1964, some 108 patients had been transferred. The kindly people of Wolsingham soon made them welcome and although the wards were old huts, they were brightened up and redecorated and were quite an improvement when compared to the gross degrading overcrowding at Winterton. Dr Duggan Keen, and especially Dr Ada Glynn were responsible for the care of the patients and the staff rapidly adjusted to the new situation.

In 1966 the water supply again caused problems, this time the water was contaminated by too many germs. The pathology laboratory at Bishop Auckland General Hospital had routinely been examining the purity of the water and though no particular disease had yet occurred, it was highly likely that soon an epidemic would develop. All water used for drinking had to be boiled and the collecting tanks drained and sterilised. The private moor supply from the springs was cut off and water supplied from the Durham County Water Board.

There had also been, for some years problems with sewage — a narrow pipe had been installed in the lane leading from the hospital but often was blocked and the road flooded, but perhaps with the change of type of patient and reduction of the operating sessions, this seems to have abated and was not mentioned in the Minutes after 1966.

Mr Richards retired in 1972 after 24 years service as Administration Assistant for the hospitals in the dales. The number of beds allocated to Newcastl General Hospital was increased to 20 and now two operating sessions were held per week, but anaesthetic problems gradually grew worse and the beds, instead of being used for short term relatively simple surgical cases became used for long term serious surgical, often incurable and dying patients, and this threw great strain on the nursing staff. The future of the surgical unit became doubtful but it continued until June, 1977, when the unit was closed.

Drs Rutter and Goodall were now in charge of the psychiatric patients and they organised a household unit to teach some of the patients household skills so that they could be taught how to live outside the hospital and in June, 1977, the unit was operating with six patients in residence.

By that year the overcrowding at Winterton was beginning to diminish and the District Management Team were determined to remove it altogether. It gradually became apparent that eventually the beds at Winterton and Sedgefield General Hospital together with the new units at Darlington, Durham and North Tees would be sufficient, and that the psychiatric beds at Holywood would become unnecessary. Furthermore the fabric of the huts was deteriorating — most were first World War wooden huts. The length of time needed to close Holywood was unknown but 8 - 10 years was mentioned. There were 105 psychiatric beds in use in 1979.

In 1983 it was stated that closure of Holywood would save £710,000 per year but there was a mounting campaign against the closure by the psychiatric nurses and local authorities and others and this occupied some newspaper space. Cuts in manpower in the Health Service made nationally, in November, 1983, led to the closure of two wards and the number of available psychiatric beds fell to 86 and by March, 1985, when the official consultation process to close the hospital began there were only 49 patients (including four General Practitioner beds). The buildings — mainly the huts, were decaying and the Hall itself could not really be used for patients. Essential maintenance was becoming more difficult and more expensive. Much capital work would be needed to bring the hospital up to a reasonable standard. Even then the difficulties of visiting and shortage of staff and particularly expert ancillary staff would continue.

In 1985 the Regional Health Authority agreed to the closure of Holywood. There were now only 33 patients and despite a last appeal from the Community Health Council to the Minister of Health, the hospital closed on 19th July, 1986. The four General Practitioner beds were transferred to Horn Hall Hospital and the remaining, 16 psychiatric patients were taken to Sedgefield Community Hospital. A few weeks later the Community Health Council reported that they found the patients had settled quite happily in their new surroundings.

Winterton Hospital

Winterton Hospital originally known as the County Lunatic Asylum was built in 1857. The county justices, responsible then for pauper lunatics had proposed to build it in 1827, but then decided the time was not expedient. However, in 1855 they began to buy land near Sedgefield and after 52 acres had been acquired, started to build and by 1857 sufficient building had been done to allow reception of some patients. Further land purchases continued and eventually the site consisted of 350 acres and included at one time, three farms. The first medical superintendent — Dr Smith — was appointed in June 1857. Originally the patients were transferred to Winterton from Bath Lane Institution which was an overflow asylum for patients from Bensham Hospital in Gateshead. Building, of course, continued as the patients arrived and it was thought that they could help by planting seeds, and preparing the grounds of the new hospital.

By October, 1859, 131 men and 120 women patients were in residence. The justices inspected the premises and found "prints were bought for the wards and the changed environment had already produced a more cheerful demeanour in the patients". These patients were only admitted to hospital by order of the magistrates. A relieving officer, or later, a duly authorised officer, who saw the patient, called one or two doctors to examine the patient to certify that he or she was a danger to themselves, or to others and was in need of hospital care. A description of the circumstances had to be recorded and then one or two magistrates from a panel, were called by the authorised officer to see the patient. If the magistrate agreed then the forms were completed and the patient was removed to Winterton.

Some doctors resented the interposition of a magistrate and were very glad when the requirement was abolished in the 1950's. Yet in many cases, if the magistrates were interested, it was very helpful to have an outside opinion, as it was always unpleasant and worrying to have to deprive a person of his or her liberty, perhaps indefinitely.

The law stated that if the order was made and was legally correct, Winterton had to accept the patient. The law did not however, say anything about the state or staffing of Winterton and the inability to control admissions bedevilled the hospital and became the major problem. Severe overcrowding is the main theme of this account.

The minute books of the hospital from 1857 to 1948 are held in the Durham County Public Records Department but I felt that I should concentrate only on the hospital in the last 40 years — the period when it came under the control of the National Health Service.

Each major psychiatric hospital had its own Hospital Management Committee. These psychiatric hospitals were quite different from the voluntary hospitals which really only dealt with short term acute illness and were also different from the Poor Law Hospitals. The psychiatric hospitals were often in isolated areas. The patients usually under legal detention —

though some hospitals were experimenting with informal or voluntary admissions and Cherry Knowle Hospital at Ryhope, Sunderland had one such ward for male and female patients in 1937 but this was quite exceptional. The grounds of the hospital were usually large and so was the hospital. Usually several hundred patients were in residence — in Winterton some two thousand. Many of the patients remained for life. There were workshops for the patients and the hospital campus contained houses for the staff including medical staff.

Treatment was limited, cure rare, and the aim was mainly to provide custodial care under secure conditions. Wards and departments were always kept locked and moving from ward to ward by the staff needed constant use of keys.

One of the first actions of the Hospital Management Committee at its inaugural meeting in July, 1948, was to order that male nurses should not be responsible for cleaning all the windows. It was agreed that one of the duties of the nurse was to make the immediate environment of the patient clean and bright and tidy and therefore the windows immediately around the patient would continue to be cleaned by the male nurses. They would however, no longer clean all windows above ground level, or windows in corridors, passages, houses, flats, the church and administrative buildings. The committee appointed two window cleaners.

By August 1948 there were 1985 patients, just over half were female — 1011. The visiting committee inspected the female wards in the main building (many were held in other buildings) and said they were very pleased with everything. I assume that the dormitories were empty and the patients usually at that time, got up and wandered round the grounds, sat in the day rooms or worked in various parts of the hospital.

The minutes of the day were somewhat discursive but not very informative. One of the main reports was the very long list of staff who had taken short term absence from duty. The names, position held, dates of the period off work and the reason given were listed and 3 - 4 foolscap sheets were usually needed each fortnight for this purpose. No comment was ever made about the length of the list or its contents. I turned these pages over quickly, but on one occasion noted that one of the male artisan staff had taken four hours off one day. The reason "to get married". I wondered which part of the day he had come into work.

The psychiatric hospitals were all inspected regularly by the Commissioner of the Board of Control in London. Usually two visitors came. They had the right to visit at any time, but usually did warn the hospital. They came to see the patients were properly looked after, that the detention orders were legally correct and because they visited many hospitals they could sometimes informally mention developments in other institutions which appeared to be helpful. They could not issue orders. They reported to their Board of Control about the things they had seen and sent a copy of the report to the Hospital Management Committee. However, only extracted comments appeared in the Committee Minutes.

At Winterton for several years, with one exception, the same two visitors always came. They wrote eloquent, tactful reports and usually praised the staff. The report in 1949 was a little more precise. They said that the buildings at Winterton were old fashioned and scattered. They were overcrowded and there was a general lack of space. There was a shortage of female nursing staff but everyone was trying to overcome the handicaps and all concerned were entitled to congratulations. There were 1997 patients and at night overcrowding amounted to 165 men and 97 women. Overcrowding was most noticeable in the sick and infirm wards.

The Commissioners noted that new buildings were contemplated and that the Hospital Management Committee had recommended to the Regional Hospital Board new sick and infirm wards be built (I have not seen any minute to this effect). The Commissioners felt there was need for a bigger entertainments hall and a new nurses' home — a number of nurses of both sexes still had to sleep in rooms adjacent to the wards.

There were 41 imbecile children in one ward who should, the Commissioners said, be removed to Aycliffe Hospital.

They also mentioned that at that time Winterton was essentially in four parts — a modern reception hospital, some outlying buildings for both sexes, the main building and another big block previously known as Winterton. There were no plans to modernise these latter two buildings but provision of sanitary annexes, improved accommodation and provision of modern facilities stood out as in need of attention.

The day staff consisted of 236 men all whole-time and 115 whole-time female nurses with 69 part-time female. The night staff was 24 men and 22 women.

The extension of central heating, and equipment needing electricity were dependent on hospital boilers and engineering plant which needed modernisation. The post mortem room also should be modernised. The Commissioners said that following one short visit they could not detail all the changes needed.

The start of the National Health Service revealed the poor standards of buildings, shortage of staff and often squalid conditions provided for long term sick patients — the physically ill, the elderly, the mentally defective and the psychiatric patients. This was found all over the country and Durham was no exception. It seemed that once such patients had been removed from the community, the community forgot about them. Most doctors and hospital consultants never saw inside these buildings.

Some councils and management committees when they came into being managed to improve things slowly, many could not, and some did not appear to try very hard. It was clear that throughout the country there was an enormous task and the post war shortages made it certain that change would only occur slowly. Winterton was no exception, but as the largest psychiatric hospital in the region, its problems were proportionately greater.

However, in the late 1940's there was more active treatment of psychiatric patients. Electro-convulsive therapy replaced the production of fits by chemical means and still later the addition of muscle relaxants abolished the risk of fractures during the treatment. Insulin coma therapy for schizophrenia was widely tried. Leucotomy — dividing some fibres in the brain surgically was being attempted and was thought to help some obsessive symptoms. Although these treatments were later often abandoned and replaced by special drugs, they seemed at the time to be helpful and they gave the staff and the patients hope.

The Management Committee wrote to the Regional Board in August 1950, about the overcrowding. "The Committee are strongly of the opinion that the most stressing and urgent need of the hospital, is that some immediate steps be taken to relieve the excessive overcrowding now taking place. The Committee are gravely concerned over the very low standard of accommodation which they can offer to their patients and consider that such circumstances under which the patients are forced to live are prejudicial to their physical well being and certainly cannot be beneficial to their mental treatment. The Hospital Management therefore urgently request the Regional Hospital Board to take immediate steps to alleviate the position either by the provision of a building for chronic patients or as a treatment centre".

A reply was received in November, but the minutes do not record the details.

The shortage of female staff became more severe and despite the General Nursing Councils ruling that staff should be at least 18 years old, girls of 16½ were taken on for nursing duties. There were still 34 mentally defective children in the hospital and the usual number of patients.

Dr McGilp the Medical Superintendent retired in November, 1953, and was succeeded by Dr G.E. Duggan-Keen. In the same year the Board of Control Commissioners visited the hospital. These two were not the usual visitors. They made some clear and astringent comments but unfortunately they never returned and the previous two Commissioners continued to visit and give kindly bland reports. They invariably gave a great deal of praise but failed, in my view, to say clearly what they found and what was wrong. Such clarity, if it had been attempted, might have assisted the members of the Management Committee who were trying to improve the conditions.

In 1953 the hospital laundry service was breaking down. Mr Leslie Bird came down from the Regional Hospital Board and issued a scathing report, gradually learned to live with it. Alterations to the wards, and redecoration all were occurring. Although the actual number of beds was reduced, there were now more types of treatment available and new drugs to use. These together with the increased movement of patients, and the presence of workmen in and around the wards worsened the effects of industrial action and the staff were in fact, under greater pressure, despite fewer patients. Over all this was the great difficulty, with the long serving staff of coping with the idea of change itself. The staff, like all those in similar hospitals — large enclosed units — had lived almost in a world of their own and working practices had become rather rigid. It was time, even late, for change but it could not be and was not, easy.

One effect of industrial "action" was to help the hospital. By restricting admissions, the union quickened the rate of the removal of beds.

There were still areas of overcrowding, lack of privacy and lockers and personalised clothing. The number of nurses was still too low and some long stay wards had only one nurse per duty per shift. The Neville sector dealing with Bishop Auckland together with also the Hartlepool sector were still overcrowded and had 79 more patients than they were recommended by Dr Bringan. The Neville sector had 357 patients scattered over 15 wards but really only one 30 bedded ward was for acute cases, to serve a population of 115,000.

In November, 1979, Dr Duggan Keene who had been so active as Medical Superintendent and helpful at Bishop Auckland in the earlier years and later at Durham, and of course, always at Winterton, became ill and soon it was clear that he would have to retire on health grounds.

The forensic psychiatry unit was active and had 18 adolescent boys in 1981. Dr Westbury wanted further facilities for girls and also for adults. However, as he had indicated that he would shortly retire it was decided to defer a decision on these two proposals.

By November, 1981, the number of beds had been reduced to 1063 — only ten above the figure suggested by Dr Bringan. The special small team of officers at Winterton composed of an Administrator, the Director of Nursing Services and a Consultant Psychiatrist had planned the reduction of beds by the District Management Team and the Area Health Authority. Despite all the difficulties and complaints and sometimes bitter opposition, the plan had been, at last, carried out successfully.

The District Health Authority Takes Over

A new reorganisation of the Health Service was under way, the Area Health Authority was to be abolished, and the District Health Authority started on 1st April, 1982.

From 1982 — not because of the appearance of the new District Authority however, psycho-geriatrics became the fashionable concept. Geriatrics as a speciality had evolved in the early years of the Health Service to deal with the disclosed demand for adequate care for the elderly housed in bad conditions, and often neglected. Now the geriatric wards were full of confused elderly patients. A large number of similar patients occupied beds in psychiatric hospitals. Both the geriatricians and the psychiatrists wanted to concentrate on more acute types of illness. Psycho-geriatrics as a term was invented. To the geriatrician this meant care must be given by the psychiatrist in his beds, to the psychiatrist it meant the geriatrician was responsible.

The suggested solution was to appoint psycho-geriatric consultants. They would look after the elderly confused patients — now called elderly severe mentally infirm — of course reduced to the initials ESMI. The numbers of such patients in the community was rising because more people were living to the age when they could become demented. This increase is likely to continue. However, one good result of the recognition of the problem has been the increase in the study of the causes of this illness and exploration of possible methods of prevention or remotely, of cure. In the past senile dementia was recognised but regarded as inevitable. Now new clinics had to be developed and some beds made available and more help sought from the community.

Child psychiatry was also becoming more prominent. No proposals to use Winterton for these children were made but a unit at Darlington was developed and out-patient facilities provided at Bishop Auckland. A travelling day hospital for psychiatric patients was started by Dr Rutter and Dr Goodall in Crook and later extended to Bishop Auckland in 1982.

Further industrial action in 1982 restricted psychiatric admissions to emergencies only. Later in the same year a scheme for staff to suggest improvements at Winterton was begun and there were rewards to staff who made suggestions for improvement of the care of patients.

Psycho-surgery and electro convulsive therapy were in sharp decline. Indeed the surgery had ceased by May, 1975. At last in 1983 the squalid post mortem room at Winterton was closed and any necessary examinations were carried out in the upgraded mortuary at Bishop Auckland. Physical restraint by harness and padded rooms were now things of the past. The greater space around the patients, better and safer drugs had greatly improved the care of the patients.

Alcoholism was recognised as a growing problem and one consultant took special interest in this. He admitted patients to Winterton for treatment but this of course put greater pressure on the small number of acute beds. A behavioural therapy unit of 16 beds and a rehabilitation unit of 26 beds were established.

Clearly in the last few years Winterton has changed. It was being moved from being mainly an institution for custodial care, possibly for life to a more active centre for treatment. Yet, although the tendency was to say nearest their home. A few days after delivery the baby and mother return to Winterton and treated as if they were at home — the Community Midwife attends and the resident nursing staff care for her psychiatric needs and look after the baby with Paediatric Consultant help if needed. The unit can handle four mothers and babies at a time and if necessary until the baby is almost a year old. In many cases the reason for admission is post-natal depression. The small rooms and quietness and the efficiency and interest of the nursing staff make this an excellent unit, further improved by allowing fathers to visit baby and mother almost any time to fit their work.

These transformations have been carried out in the last ten years against a background of industrial action on a national scale, financial stringency and several reorganisations of the administrative staff. Over the same period some critics announced that the National Health Service was in the early stages of decay!

The Resurgence of the former Hospitals for Infectious Diseases

As I have mentioned, the infectious diseases hospitals in Bishop Auckland, Spennymoor and Stanhope were all closed. The smallpox hospital at Binchester was used for mentally subnormal women and then demolished. The Sedgefield Isolation Hospital became part of Winterton Hospital.

Three hospitals remained — Helmington Row, Tindale Crescent and Horn Hall. Leazes Hospital had ceased to admit tuberculosis patients and then was used for young chronic sick, convalescent and General Practitioner patients but was then closed and eventually taken over by Durham County Council.

Helmington Row Hospital near Crook had fever beds in three wards and one long narrow ward had a balcony alongside the long wall. This was a ward for advanced cases of tuberculosis. Dr Fenwick Lishman was Medical Superintendent when the hospital was used for infectious diseases. In 1950 he enthusiastically supported the change to the care of the elderly. One ward was altered and redecorated and took some patients from the overcrowded chronic sick wards at the General Hospital. With the experience of the appalling conditions in Blocks 2 and 3 at the General Hospital everyone was determined to try to provide spacious clean and odour free accommodation. Money was in short supply and the actual work of altering the buildings was often carried out by the maintenance staff at the hospital. This meant they were unable to keep up with normal repair and maintenance work and this naturally caused problems.

Yet Mr Luxford insisted that if this was not done no improvements in the chronic sick situation could be expected for years ahead. Gradually the Regional Hospital Board was able to contribute some money so that contractors could be brought in. However, the changes were restricted and the large stoves in the entrance hall of each ward and the stoves in the two halves of each ward had to remain for several years. Helmington Row

Hospital was renamed Homelands Hospital. Later a start was made in converting Tindale Crescent Hospital for use for the chronic sick elderly patients.

Branches of the League of Friends were formed at each hospital and the members gave great help both by raising funds and supplying extra comforts and also by joining with other organisations to assist in taking some patients on outings.

Early in the development of the hospitals we felt there was a need to provide side wards with room for two beds so that married couples could be admitted and share one room. However, we discovered that this was not very satisfactory. There were many fewer applications for admission than we had expected, usually elderly couples deteriorate at different rates and even if both are partly disabled they can often manage with community help. From time to time we found the couple did not want to share a room. On once occasion a chair bound woman was observed to drop something on the floor. She then ordered her husband — who was more mobile than she was — to bend down an pick it up. As he did so she gave him a push. He fell and was injured. Later she repeated this trick. He was greatly relieved when we separated them.

There was a continuing shortage of ancillary staff such as Physiotherapists, Occupational Therapists, Chiropodists and Social Workers. Consultant Geriatricians with adequate training in the new specialty were rare and despite advertisements an personal contacts, no appointment could be made for several years. However, the wards were steadily improved and by 1975 became something of a show place in North East England. The coke stoves in the wards were removed, central heating was installed and after a lot of argument the stoves in the entrance halls were also removed. Previously it had been feared that this might cause the roof to give way. This did not happen and the entrance to each ward was vastly improved. New side wards and a variety of day rooms allowed more dispersal of the patients and more room. Each of the two hospitals had around 80 beds and although there was always and continues to be, a shortage of nurses, the majority of nurses were very loyal and took great pride in the running of their hospital and the fact that they got to know their patients very well. Many patients were admitted often from other hospitals and were able to improve and go home. Others were admitted for a week or two to give relatives a rest and then went home again. Of course age cannot be denied and some patients died. If several deaths occurred in a short time it was important to defer admission for a few days to allow the nurses and other staff to grieve because they became inevitably, deeply attached to their patients.

Occasionally it is said of geriatric units "that you only go there to die". In fact it is in acute medical units especially with coronary care units that the majority of deaths occur. It is a function of a good geriatric unit, as of all hospitals, to provide for the dying patient. Both the patient and the relatives must be given proper care, pain and discomfort relieved, senseless and useless medical and surgical interference avoided, tests with no likely benefit to the patient stopped, and support to the relatives maintained. In all these respects the geriatric services in South West Durham provide a good caring environment.

Visiting hours were steadily extended and now, as in the childrens wards, are quite free — some relatives call in on the way to work in the morning, others come at lunch-time, in the afternoons and evenings. Whereas in the old Blocks 2 and 3 at the General Hospital almost no patient was ever visited, now it is very rare for a single patient in the hospital not to have a visitor.

The old laundry buildings at each hospital were converted into social areas where occupational therapy, games and discussion groups can take place. The Manpower Services Commission have provided two young women to help provide these services and they told me recently that they are enjoying this work.

The appointment of Dr Bernard Walsh in 1981 with his great enthusiasm gave great impetus to the service and when he left to go to Dublin his successors Dr R.W.G. Prescott and Dr A. Mehrzad have continued the improvements with enthusiastic support for the staff.

Horn Hall

When Horn Hall ceased admitting tuberculosis patients, for a time it was used to care for ambulant male chronic sick patients, some male convalescents from various hospitals on Tyne and Wearside and for four patients under the care of General Practitioners. However, the unit of 21 beds was too small for such a variety. The ambulant chronic sick deteriorated and soom became bedridden, the word convalescent was misused. Some Surgeons finding the patient had inoperable and incurable cancer sent the patient forty or fifty miles from home to "convalesce" at Horn Hall. Some of these patients died within days — some even within hours, of admission. The convalescent beds were closed by the Regional Hospital Board, the four General Practitioner beds remained and all the rest of the beds used for chronic sick men. The physical difficulties of caring for these men on a split level site and with a few patients upstairs in the main old Hall with difficult steps and levels made care and supervision very difficult indeed. As elsewhere there were severe staff shortages but again the loyalty and hardwork of the small staff was remarkable.

In the last two years alterations to the old Hall now 250 - 290 years old, have allowed the beds upstairs to be closed and all the patients to be nursed on the ground floor or to sleep in the riverside block. The decor and bed spacing has been improved. The number of General Practitioner beds has been increased to eight and the whole area is animated, cheerful and charming.

In all three hospitals overall supervision is by the Consultants in geriatric medicine and they arrange admissions and discharges. The day to day care is provided by one General Practitioner in each hospital. This has been the case since the hospitals were used for geriatric patients and has had great advantages. Dr John Anderson and then Dr D.T. Prescott then Dr McManners and Dr Bolton have in turn worked at Tindale Cresent, whilst at Homelands Hospital Dr Fenwick Lishman was succeeded by Dr G. Ferguson. At Horn Hall Dr D. Thomson and his Partners and then after retirement, their successors in the practice have carried out the work. The partners of these doctors covered in emergencies or holidays. The doctors often knew the patient at home and certainly knew the district from which the patient came and frequently had relatives of the patient as their own patient. They thus could supply an accurate background of knowledge of the previous history and social conditions which were and is invaluable. Even very keen cohorts of junior hospital doctors, changing each six months cannot bring this special knowledge and experience to the care of the patient.

The units have become friendly and home like with a relaxed atmosphere not easily achievable in an acute general hospital ward.

Binchester Whins Hospital

I have mentioned this hospital built on the windy plateau for smallpox patients. By 1948 it was clear that it was unlikely to be used again for smallpox and for a time it stood empty. Shortly after the Management Committee took over Dr Raine suggested to the Committee that space could be created at the General Hospital by moving some 41 mentally defective patients — all women — from the General Hospital to Binchester Whins. The Regional Board was asked to approve this but Ministry of Health approval was needed to close down a smallpox unit. In December, 1949, approval was obtained and early in 1950 the patients were moved from Block 4 to Binchester. There were two parallel dormitories and at one end another hut used as day room, dining room, staff quarters and a small kitchen and storage areas.

The patients all lived together for many years. Many had been in institutions since childhood, one woman had been admitted because she was pregnant, unmarried and defective. Her baby was born in the General Hospital and later joined her mother in the little colony and now at the age of 19 was in Binchester with her mother.

In December, 1950, Dr Raine died and I was instructed by the Regional Hospital Board to take over the post of Medical Superintendent at Binchester as the law required such a post to be filled. There was no salary attached to the post however! All the patients were under legal detention. Mrs Sands was in charge of the nursing care.

As a result of a High Court case in which it was decided that the patients already detained in a psychiatric unit could not be recertified at the intervals the law demanded, on the grounds that they needed care and protection, when clearly by virtue of being in hospital they already received that protection, the legal status of thousands of patients had to be reviewed. Unless other grounds for ordering the continued detention could be put forward, the patient had to be freed from the order. They could now be discharged, take their own discharge or remain in hospital as "informal" patients. At Binchester it was decided that all the patients would now be informal. None sought to leave — they had nowhere to go and most had no relations.

At times fighting would occur, often between the mother and daughter; I would be summoned during the night to find them trying to pull each others hair. Gradually it became apparent that the daughter, though unable to read or write, was not in fact mentally subnormal. We managed to get her employment with the help of social workers in North Yorkshire. She managed quite well and after a year or two became engaged to be married. We had no legal authority to interfere but she kept us informed and cooperated with the social workers and after enquiries, we felt she would be able to manage, a cottage was found and she was married. A year or two later she visited Binchester bringing her first baby, beautifully clothed, spotlessly clean and delightful. Later she asked if she could take her mother to live with them. We were reluctant to agree — but had no legal means of stopping this. However, we arranged visits for a few days, then extended visits. All seemed to go well and finally mother was discharged to live with the daughter and her husband and for some years we heard from them and all was well.

Other patients were also found work in the community and a few eventually discharged. Others worked in Bishop Auckland General Hospital. When the question of discharge was raised we proceeded very slowly before agreeing. Some would call this paternalistic behaviour. It was. Yet it seemed right and proper to be concerned about women who had been in institutions for most if not all of their life.

As patients were discharged or died they were replaced by transfers from Aycliffe Hospital. One condition imposed was that the new patient should be a non smoker. None of the existing patients had ever smoked. There was considerable risk of fire. One small fire did in fact occur in some straw outside the building. The fire brigade arrived and in those days had difficulty in getting enough water to deal adequately with the outbreak.

The nursing staff were all assistant nurses. They carried out their duties quietly and calmly, with good humour and kindness. The hospital was isolated and in winter in those early years the roads easily became blocked with snow. The staff often then, had to stay overnight in makeshift beds and on one occasion had to stay almost a week. At that time I could not get my car to the hospital, the main Bishop Auckland to Spennymoor road was blocked and I went along the riverside to beyond Binchester Hall and thence had to walk knee deep in the snow over the fields. From time to time the electricity supply failed as it was supplied from one of the collieries. A supply of lamps and torches was always to hand.

Visitors to the patients were rare — perhaps three or four per year, but members of the local community came in from time to time to help. Bus trips for the patients were organised and the local bus drivers were always most helpful in getting the patients in and out. An annual holiday for most of the patients was held at Marske holiday camp run by the YMCA until the condition of the huts there made it impossible to continue. For a few years other venues were used but gradually as the patients became older and more disabled, fewer were able to go.

The land around the hospital became subject to opencast coal removal. For a time the hospital was surrounded by the large machinery. We did ask the coal owners (with tongue in cheek) to demolish the hospital to get at the coal underneath and pay for its restoration elsewhere. We did not succeed.

In 1978 the patients were moved to Sedgefield General Hospital where two wards had been carefully altered to make very attractive residential units. These were certainly much better than those at Binchester, despite the changes that had been made there over the years. The patients now had access to occupational therapy and other facilities and rapidly settled down in their new environment. Some of the staff at Binchester went with the patients, other retired. The patients were made very welcome by the Sedgefield Hospital and the community around. No new admissions were to be accepted and at the time of writing the numbers have fallen to 21.

A Note on the Other Hospitals within the District

Sedgefield General Hospital

I have made only passing reference to Sedgefield Community Hospital. It was built almost alongside Winterton Hospital during the 1939-45 War as an Emergency Medical Service Hospital. When the War ended it became a General Hospital with 319 beds under the control of North Tees Hospital Management Committee and hence I have not attempted to trace its detailed history.

In the first few years of the Health Service consideration was given to the suggestion that the hospital should be used for long stay surgical tuberculosis patients — people with bone and joint tuberculosis especially, but with the advent of streptomycin and the reduction of milk borne tuberculosis the suggestion was abandoned and the hospital continued as a General Hospital with out-patient facilities. There was no Maternity Unit. As the new North Tees Hospital was built and reorganisation of the Health Service in 1974 occurred, the hospital was transferred to Durham Area Health Authority and the South West Durham Health District. When North Tees Hospital was eventually opened, closure of the Sedgefield Hospital was suggested by the Regional Health Authority.

This suggestion was met by tremendous local opposition and the hospital remained open and was called Sedgefield Community Hospital. By 1977 a new geriatric day unit was opened and a ward of 15 beds was allocated for use by General Practitioners, and as mentioned in the account of Binchester Whins, two wards were converted to provide excellent accommodation for the 33 women from that hospital.

In 1980 a temporary building at Winterton used for the elderly women had deteriorated and become dangerous. The patients were therefore transferred to Sedgefield Community Hospital and two years later funds were allocated by the Regional Health Authority to Winterton to rebuild three male wards and a dormitory housing 90 men in squalid overcrowded conditions. There wasn't room to put a small chair between the beds. These wards had caused great concern to the Management Team at Winterton and they immediately evacuated the patients to Sedgefield Community Hospital. The changes effected in these overcrowded wards and dormitory are mentioned at the end of the account of Winterton Hospital.

All this put pressure on the Sedgefield Community Hospital and many people felt these patients would not return to Winterton and there was considerable concern. However, as planned, the refurbishing of the Winterton wards was completed and the patients returned to the new excellent wards.

The new psychogeriatric unit at Sedgefield Community Hospital had been developed by conversion of a unit used for aministrative staff. It provides a delightful spacious unit for 10 in-patients and around 80 day patients per week. These latter patients are brought to the hospital by minibus early in the morning and returned home late in the afternoon. Two nurses go from the unit with the bus to collect the patients. This has great benefits because the nurses see the relatives, learn of the latest problems and can see the type of home to which the patient returns and on return can tell the relatives of the happenings in the day unit. This enables the nurses, patients and relatives to see each others problems in a direct way almost unknown in most hospitals and the nurse in charge of the ward when I visited recently was delighted and enthusiastic about the arrangements. The patients are greeted on arrival with tea and toast. The ward provides all the usual facilities — occupation therapy, aids to daily living and must be one of the brightest and best in North East England.

Lady Eden Hospital, Bishop Auckland

This Hospital was built nearly ninety years ago to commemorate Queen Victoria's Long reign. It was built as a result of the persistent efforts of Lady Sybil Eden (Lord Avon's Mother) who together with a nucleus of enthusiastic supporters, devoted much time and energy and money towards the establishment of the Hospital, which in the course of time formed an integral part of Bishop Auckland and its industry.

When the scheme was first mooted the Committee experienced the vicissitudes of fortune. There were doubts and apprehension in many peoples minds as to whether a small town like Bishop Auckland could afford to maintain a Hospital, let alone defray the cost of building one. Not many held the opinion that the town with its population of only 11,000 could support a scheme of this nature. The miners, after some initial uncertainty, were sufficiently farsighted to endorse it, and gave a generous offer of support.

From the onset the Committee ploughed a lone furrow, listened to criticism with calm philosophy, and decided to carry on with the determination which earned them the everlasting gratitude of a generous hearted public. The majority of the pioneers have now long since shuffled off this mortal coil, but their spirit still lives in a town which benefitted greatly from their wisdom and self sacrifice and I presume that our present day League of Friends, and in particular the support of the recent Scanner Appeal is a newer generation of the same sort of people.

Similarly Lady Eden with initiative and enterprise visualised the benefits to be derived from a hospital which could cater for even a small number of in-patients and she did much valuable spade work before the first Committee was actually formed. At a meeting held in the Temperance Hall (now the Masonic Hall in Victoria Street, Bishop Auckland) on 26th March, 1897, with the Lord Bishop of Durham in the Chair, it was decided to collect funds to establish a Cottage Hospital for the Auckland District and a Committee was formed with Lady Eden as President, the Joint Honorary Secretaries were Dr T.A. McCullagh and Mr J.H. Duff and Dr M. Wardle was a Member of the Committee.

It was felt that there was no more suitable way in which the sixty years reign of Queen Victoria could be celebrated than by providing a place where the numerous accidents which were continually taking place in the collieries and works of the neighbourhood could be treated. No such place existed at the time and injuries which were not treated at home almost invariably had to be sent to Newcastle upon Tyne.

It is of some interest to note that subscriptions already promised to Lady Eden at that time:- Bolkow Vaughan and Co., £200; North Bitchburn Coal Co. Ltd., £100; Ecclesiastical Commissioners, £100; Pease and Partners, £100; The Bishop of Durham £50; Lord Eldon £50; Lord Barnard £50; Lord Boyne, £10; and the Duchess of Cleveland, £10. Shortly after this list had been circulated, subscriptions began to come in rapidly and on the 20th July, 1897, the following letter was sent out to the Miners Lodges in the area:-

Dear Sir

As the subscription fund to the building fund of the Lady Eden Cottage Hospital already amounts to more than £1,300 the Members of the Committee feel that the time has arrived when something definite should be ascertained as to the share your Colliery is willing to contribute towards the support of the Institution.

It is anticipated that the annual sum required for the maintenance of eight beds and of the Resident Nurse and Servant will be £400.

If the Members of your Lodge desire any further information the Committee will be glad to send a deputation to address them and to discuss the scheme in details.

We are your Obedient Servants.

T.A. McCullagh
J.H. Duff
HONORARY SECRETARIES

It is interesting to note that at that time the Northern Echo, The Times and The Herald were asked for their generous support of the scheme.

The Voluntary Committee pressed ahead with their plan; the Ecclesiastical Commissioners having been asked to donate a site opposite the Auckland Workhouse in South Road, as it was then called. In December, 1897, they replied refusing to give this site but sold it, at a reduced price of £150. Two Architects were asked to submit plans, the proposed building to be adjudicated by Sir Henry Bardell. Following this tenders were to be invited. In April, 1898, the Committee met in the Town Hall, Bishop Auckland, when tenders were opened and examined, a tender of £1,557.18 produced by a combination of local firms, was accepted.

The foundation stone of the Hospital was laid by the fourth Earl Grey, who was Lady Eden's cousin, (a monument to the first Earl Grey is Grey's Monument in Newcastle upon Tyne) on the 23rd July, 1898, and the stone to this effect can be seen on the front of the building at the present, and the Hospital was duly opened by the Right Honourable, The Earl of Roseberry, (the former Liberal Prime Minister) on the 8th September, 1898, and the following Notice was sent out by the Secretaries; "as you are doubtless aware the Right Honourable, The Earl of Roseberry has consented to open the Hospital on the 8th September, 1898. In order that as many inhabitants as possible may be present, it has been decided to commence the Ceremony at 6.00 p.m. The Committee earnestly requests that you will attend in large numbers to welcome the distinguished Statesman, who is making his first public visit to this district".

The first patient was admitted on the 22nd September, 1899, from that date to the 3rd June, 1900, 34 In-patients received treatment. In addition 25 cases of injury had been treated as Out-Patients. The injuries had not been sufficiently severe to need detention in the wards.

A Nurse Blume had been appointed as Matron, out of a shortlist of five, at £40 per annum. Shortly after protestations by Mr J.T. Rudd (a family connected with Spoors, of Bishop Auckland and Dressers of Darlington) this small salary was raised to £60 per annum. It is interesting to note certain items from the maintenance account from 22nd September, 1899, to

15th June, 1900, and certainly interesting to compare them with present day prices. Provisions, £75.7s.9d.; coal, £20.15s.8d.; uniforms, £13.12s.; drugs, £17.5s.5d.; and furniture £30. In all the total maintenance account for nine months was only £255.

Not long after the opening of the Hospital the question of enlarging the building arose (a situation not uncommon with any of the present day buildings) and this was violently opposed by the various Miners Lodges who were in the opinion that the Hospital was large enough. However, at a Governors Meeting held on the 7th January, 1904, a draft agreement for the purchase of new land was produced and in March, of that year the land was purchased.

In spite of difficulties and considerable opposition against the enlargements scheme, the Hospital progressed to the satisfaction of all concerned with its welfare, and in due course those opposed to the scheme became whole-heartedly in favour of it. It is on record, however, that the Members of the General Committee, House Committee and Board of Governors did not always see eye to eye on administrative matters, but criticism being good for the soul difficulties were ironed out, and fractured spirits calmed and friction gradually erased, (not much different from what happens today). Records state that later in the year a new Ward was added, which accommodated seven beds, and increased accommodation was also provided for the nursing staff.

In 1910 a suggestion for X-Ray apparatus was mentioned, but the Committee held that the time was inopportune to go to the expense of installing the apparatus and further consideration was deferred to a later date.

In the years between the two World Wars difficulties arose with regard to money raising schemes to keep pace with ever increasing costs of administration, maintenance and other charges. It was during these years that many revenue producing concerns went out of existence, chiefly the collieries in and around Bishop Auckland, the closing of which threw thousands of men out of work and thus dealt the income side of the Hospital a severe blow.

Despite this by 1930, an X-Ray apparatus had been installed and by this time a Carnival Committee had been organised in order to make a special money making effort every year. In the Summer of 1930 an Air Pageant was held at Middlestone Moor, and Miss Amy Johnson, that intrepid pioneer of solo flights to Australia, actually performed at the Air Pageant and was introduced to representatives of the Hospital Committee.

In 1932 the balance sheet showed an increase in expenditure over income for the first time, and £148 had been spent on central heating, but fortunately there were investments of about £1,000.

At this time depression in the area seemed to be at its height and through sheer necessity a Special Appeals Committee was formed. A Mr Forbes Adam had been drafted into the Bishop Auckland District to consider ways and means of helping an area which had become known as a "Distressed Area" by means of unemployment and the Appeals Committee contacted him with a view to obtaining financial assistance for the Hospital. It is not known whether or not they received any, but despite all this, the active Governors of the Hospital and many willing to help pressed ahead with plans for an extension and scores of Meetings were held to discuss this scheme, a scheme which had the blessing of many Government Officers, but never materialised. In 1936 a special announcement was made to the effect that the district was to be provided with £20,000 by the Commissioners of Special Areas to meet the Hospital needs of 130,000 inhabitants. A request for this amount and a concrete scheme for the reconstruction of the Hospital to modernise this equipment had been sent to him. The application was for £4,500 to rebuild and re-equip the present Hospital, £7,500 for extensions to include an operating theatre, £2,000 to buy, alter and furnish a detached house in the grounds adjoining for a staff hostel, £1,000 to buy and equip a motor ambulance and £5,000 for a Trustee Fund to subsidise income during the first five years of re-building. Although 3,096 out-patients attended the Hospital in 1935 the building had no Out-Patients Department, and the new scheme did provide for such facilities. Towards the middle of 1937, when there had apparently been some delay in the provision of the grant and negotiations were still going forward, it was pointed out to the Commissioner (Sir George Gillette) that the distressed areas around Bishop Auckland stood in the midst of the mining area of South West Durham, but most of the mines had been closed and trade revival could not help or bring brighter prospects to the town as many of the pits were either closed or worked out. Consequently there were only 29 collieries compared with 63 in 1923, there were over 3,000 signing on the unemployment register at Bishop Auckland Labour Exchange and over 40% of these men had been unemployed for five years or more.

Following this a 75% grant towards the cost had been approved, but the Hospital had to raise approximately £5,000 itself. A subscription list was opened and by July, 1937, donations were coming in steadily, but by this time over £1,000 had been spent on a new X-Ray apparatus.

In the late 1939's an ambulance had been purchased in blue and cream livery. The driver was a Mr Briddick. He wanted to resign because he thought it was unfair to his employer that he was away from his work so long on ambulance duties. The Committee spoke to Mr H.W. Vale a local garage proprietor, who said he was quite happy to keep Mr Briddick in his employment and also to let him continue to take the ambulance whenever necessary. The Committee decided that when the ambulance took a patient to the Royal Victoria Infirmary at Newcastle, it should wait there, if necessary 3 to 4 hours to bring the patient home again rather than make two journeys, which would incur more expense. An attempt was made to reach reciprocal agreement with the Shildon Railway Ambulance to deal with emergency cases.

It was interesting to note that on the 14th November, 1937, the Right Honourable Anthony Eden, broadcast an appeal which eventually brought in a total of over £300. From 1st February to 30th November, 1937, there was a total received or promised of £2,600 on behalf of the building fund out of £5,000 needed. At that time the Bishop Auckland Division of the British Medical Association was beginning to take some interest in the affairs of the Hospital requesting urgent improvements and enlargements, and following a letter from the then Secretary, Dr P.V. Anderson, the Governors passed the following resolution, "we agree to the provision of enlarging the Cottage Hospital (approximately thirty beds) with up-to-date appliances", and arranged for a Newcastle-upon-Tyne visiting surgeon to be made available to undertake surgical work here or elsewhere. Doctors will decide which operations are to be done here.

However, like the present day when original estimates were prepared the cost was £20,000 and after eighteen months had risen to £25,000, due to increased costs of materials, but the Commissioner had agreed to make the same grant on the higher cost as on the original, but of course, now £6,000 was needed to be raised. However, the Second World War on 3rd September, 1939 intervened and no progress was made at that time and no doubt this War had to do with the failure of the hard-working Committee to achieve its object. Between the two World Wars the medical work of this Hospital was carried out on an entirely voluntary basis by Drs Val Wardle, A.C. McCullagh and T.E. Ferguson and before them by Drs Wardle and McCullagh's fathers. During the War the complement of sixteen beds continued to function as before apart from the absence of Dr Wardle in HM Forces. After the 1939/45 War newer and younger doctors joined the Hospital staff including the return of Dr V.H. Wardle on his return from a Prisoner of War Camp in the Far East. Dr T.E. Ferguson and Dr A.C.H. McCullagh retired after long and valued service and the scheme for enlarging the Hospital was beginning to be discussed again, but with the shortage of building materials, the increased cost of building and the constant rumblings about the National Health Service nothing was done and the Hospital was in a fairly poor state of repair and decoration, and there was also a shortage of equipment. Nevertheless, attempts were made to alter the service in Bishop Auckland and Mr Monroe, the Darlington ENT Surgeon started an Out-Patient Clinic in the Hospital, and followed this in the same afternoon with an operative session of tonsils and adenoids. The X-Ray Unit was also used by the tuberculosis clinics for screening, this continued long after the commencement of the National Health Service. Dr D.B. Houston used to attend once per week and used the X-Ray Unit for screening and various examinations such as cholecystograms and barium meals.

On 5th July, 1948, on the commencement of the National Health Service, the Bishop Auckland and District Committee handed over to the Ministry of Health the Cottage Hospital at Bishop Auckland, complete with assets and investments valued at £10,000.

At the time of going to press one has sadly to report the demise of the Lady Eden Hospital as a General Practitioner Hospital after over 90 years. The South West Durham Health Authority are having to provide somewhat urgently a day unit facility in Bishop Auckland for the mentally ill and mentally handicapped and in their wisdom have decided that the Lady Eden Hospital was suitable for development as such. The Community Health Council opposed this and therefore the Regional Health Authority had to refer the matter to the Department of Health. The Minister has decided after careful consideration to agree with the South West Durham Health Authorities proposals and in consequence the General Practitioner beds are proposed to be re-located at Ward 1, Tindale Crescent Hospital and the population of Bishop Auckland will, in the early 1990s see considerable alteration and new building proceeding on the Lady Eden Hospital site.

D.T.P.

The County Maternity Home, Princes Street, Bishop Auckland (Clairmont)

The first mention of Clairmont is found in Matthew Richley's History of Auckland dated 1872, as follows:-

"Fairless Street consists of some half dozen houses on its northern side with an imposing structure called "Clairmont" opposite". (Princes Street used to be called Fairless Street and in fact at its Newgate Street end the sign of Fairless Street could be seen as recently as post 1939-45 war).

After being used as a private residence it was for some time used as a private school and eventually was converted into a Maternity Home by Durham County Council in 1921. The day to day care of maternity patients was given by local general practitioners who were called to the aid of midwives when there were obstetric problems beyond the competence of a midwife.

The County Council appointed Professor R.P. Ranken Lyle as Consultant Obstetrician and paid him 25 guineas a year plus 10 guineas per case treated together with travelling expenses of one shilling per mile. Professor Ranken Lyle was the Professor of Midwifery at Newcastle. The General Practitioners formed a rota to act as Medical Officer to the hospital and were paid. One trained nurse was appointed as Deputy Matron at £580 per year (resident), there were two Sisters at £65 per year plus £5 for night duty. Each Nursing Officer received £10 a year for uniform allowance. There was a Cook (£45), a Parlour Maid (£28), a Housemaid (£28), a Kitchen Maid (£26) and one Ward Maid (£26). All these were resident and a non resident laundress was appointed at £1 per wash plus meals daily. Some of the staff lived in Ninefields behind the hospital.

The unit remained as a General Practitioner Hospital with Consultant support, Professor Farquahar Murray succeeded Professor Ranken Lyle. In June, 1950, the hospital became a Specialist Maternity Unit under the care of Mr D.C. Galloway with 17 beds. Three beds were allocated for use by the General Practitioners. Of course by this time there also was a Maternity Unit at the General Hospital.

During the War and for years thereafter, Croxdale Hall near Durham, and Hardwick Hall near Sedgefield were used for maternity patients — the latter remained in use until the 1960's or thereabouts.

In 1973 there was a crisis in recruitment of midwives and all the patients in Clairmont were transferred to Block 3 at Bishop Auckland General Hospital together with the midwives — Clairmont was never officially closed as a Maternity Unit but was never used again. In 1974 on re-organisation of the Health Service the then Durham Area Health Authority decided it would make excellent administrative offices for South West Durham.

D.T.P.

The life of a peripheral hospital consultant in the early years of the National Health Service

Few people know much about consultants before the advent of the National Health Service. They were uncommon and worked mainly in the large teaching hospitals and there were a few — mainly surgeons, in some voluntary hospitals in the larger towns. At any time there were only eight consultant physicians in the Royal Victoria Infirmary — four senior and four assistant physicians. These consultants gave their time and knowledge free to the voluntary hospitals and earned their living by seeing private patients, some of whom would be admitted to nursing homes for surgery or medical treatment.

In the late 1930's it was becoming apparent that the days of the voluntary hospital were almost over. Costs were rising and income could not really keep pace. After the war there was a pool of young men of consultant status — chiefly in surgery or medicine, but there were many fewer in other specialties. They almost all had wide experience and often had administrative experience in the Services. They could see that some sort of National Health Service was essential, certainly as far as hospital provision went. Many not only wanted a job but wanted to move away from the central teaching hospital into what later became known as the "peripheral" hospitals, in order to build up proper modern hospital facilities and to help provide a service available to all regardless of ability to pay. I was but one of these.

When I applied for the posts there were, as was usual then, about one hundred applicants — anyone of whom could probably have done the job. The interviewing committee sat all day seeing the "short listed" candidates. Although appointed in July, 1949, the Royal Victoria Infirmary could not release me until 1st February, 1950. I was able however, to come down to Bishop Auckland one day a week from September, 1949. Like nearly all new consultant physicians of the time I had to develop a medical department, with properly equipped wards and out-patient facilities. Surgeons appointed usually had some wards recognised as surgical and an operating theatre but usually much upgrading was needed.

One important feature of the new service was the provision for seeing the patient at the patients own home. This was the domiciliary visit. These visits were made at the request of the general practitioner to the consultant concerned, for the latter to examine and advise on treatment or management of a patient who could not attend the hospital.

In addition to helping with the diagnosis and treatment, the consultant might be called to persuade a patient to enter hospital for the necessary treatment and to try to allay the fears of the patient or relatives because hospitals were strange and disturbing places. Furthermore it was widely thought that to enter a former Poor Law Hospital was a sentence of death. "You are only put in there to die" was often said to me in those early years.

I always enjoyed this domiciliary aspect of the work and invariably went with the general practitioner — indeed I can only recall three occasions in thirty years when the general practitioner was absent and this was always because of sudden illness of the doctor.

The doctor would tell me about the patient and his background and show me any relevant notes or reports. We would then go to the patients home. Most visits were in the evening, after the evening surgery had ended — usually around seven o-clock.

In the first year or two I was often shown patients with strange diseases, often congenital, in men, women and children for which nothing could be done. These were people who lived a long way from Newcastle, who could not afford a private fee and because they were not acute emergencies, could not be sent to the Royal Victoria Infirmary. Some of these diseases and malformations were only mentioned in older textbooks. The relatives were, however, grateful that a careful examination and review had been carried out and appreciated the trouble that the general practitioner had taken even though improvement was unlikely.

After a consultation, my examination completed, nearly always a bowl of warm water, soap and a clean neatly folded towel was available on a side table so that I could wash my hands. Many of the houses did not have a bathroom and many others did not have a hot water supply on tap. After about 1970 this little courtesy rarely was offered but most houses had a bathroom.

Often as the consultation ended and we were preparing to depart, the husband and wife, especially if they were elderly, would exchange a glance or a little nod. One of them would reach to the mantle shelf or under the pillow and proffer an envelope "would that be alright for your fee doctor?". It was almost always the poorest houses that this occurred. I was of course paid by the National Health Service for this visit and could not accept a private fee. I quickly learned however, to be very tactful in my refusal in order to avoid hurting the feelings of a proud and independent patient and avoid the suggestion that charity was being offered. Yet often enough a little sigh or lightening of expression suggested the relief they felt. Frequently as a compromise instead of a fee, a cup of tea and a piece of special birthday or Christmas cake was offered and gladly accepted. I was then regaled by stories of the village or past medical episodes.

One such visit took place soon after I took up my post and I didn't know the smaller roads. It was about five in the morning when the doctor rang me. He was returning to the patients house and couldn't leave her. He directed me to a road junction and assured me that a man would then redirect me. It was dark and when I slowed down for the turn, a man stepped into the roadway "Are you the doctor?" "Yes". He gave brief directions and I drove on. A mile or two later, the process was repeated. In all about five men had been strategically placed to see that I got quickly to the farm.

There were very few cars in those days and they had all walked to their appointed post.

When I arrived the doctor and I went upstairs, the family remained in the living room. As we entered the bedroom a young woman, was standing on the broad window sill about to jump into the farmyard below. The general practitioner took one arm and leg and I, the other side, and we lifted her back to bed. She was very confused and I thought she had a chronic disease of the nervous system. We injected a sedative and got her into hospital where she eventually recovered completely. This was a country practice, the general practitioner knew everyone and was able to send messages to the prospective guides knowing the instructions would be carried out. I wondered if this could have occurred in a big city.

One Friday evening after a busy day in the hospital I was asked by Dr Thomson of Stanhope to meet him and go to see a patient. I also had two other calls for the same evening. I drove to Stanhope and from there to the banks of the River Derwent between Blanchland and Edmondbyers to see the patient. We drove back over the moors. Dr Thomson returned to Stanhope but I went to Rookhope and then to the Wear Valley and over the hills south to the Tees near the road to Cauldron Snout. Then down the valley to Middleton-in-Teesdale to see Dr Dawson and his patient. From there down to Barnard Castle to Dr Pickworth and his patient. All the patients needed consultant help but none were admitted to hospital. These excellent doctors were well able to manage. It was late when I got home and it had been a long day but it had also been a beautiful summer evening, with no traffic and such a marvellous countryside that I felt a little sorry for the city consultants.

In the early years winter travelling could be trying. The boot of the car — all cars were rear wheel driven then — was weighted down with stones or a bag of sand, a spade, sacking and tow rope. A torch, old macintosh, rubber boots and old gloves were included. Some doctors told me that a pile of copies of the British Medical Journal helped the wheels to grip on the snow. Special winter tyres were fitted. I had chains but only used them once. Road clearance of snow was not as efficient as it is today and after a few hours of snow, a few inches would remain until a thaw set in — perhaps some days later. Only essential traffic used the smaller roads — a few milk vans, the postal van, an odd ambulance, the doctors car and an occasional district nurse. Few of the farmers had motorised tractors. It was important to park the car in such a way that it could be easily driven away after the visit was completed, and we usually took care to leave the car pointing downhill.

My parish grew larger, from Brandon to North Yorkshire and Northallerton, Sedgefield to Cowshill and all of Teesdale. There were weekly visits to all the hospitals in South West Durham and extra visits on demand, the General Hospital was of course visited daily and not infrequently during the night. There was also, for some years a weekly out-patient clinic at the Royal Victoria Infirmary. However, the roads though poorer than today were much less crowded. Teaching students and house officers always gave added interest to the job.

The ideas that some students had, and I think others also, that consultant physicians sat at home sipping sherry and thinking of rare esoteric diseases was far from the truth. Yet it was a satisfying life and enjoyable. At one time I thought that I had been inside at least one house in almost every street in most of the small towns and villages in the area.

My experiences were not unique and when I met colleagues, appointed around the same time as myself, and facing many of the same problems, it was quite obvious that we all lived the same sort of life.